WHAT REA

"This story is a treasure. Its value of family, knowledge, and spirituality touch the foundations of day-to-day life despite the dire circumstances within which it is set. The rich narrative plows a field that grows the reader into belonging to a distressed family and follows the author's lead in his quest to understand his tragic predicament.

"Dr. Moss's guilt, from which he refuses to absolve himself, or even allow his mother to absolve him as the offended party, has Shakespearean qualities. The quest for the stroke's cause and potential cure provides a powerful education to the reader on the mechanics of bloodstream disease. The byplay between god and science, serendipity and plaque, is fascinating.

"The devastating effect that Matilda's stroke has on her son endures throughout the story. Flashback scenes provide a rich tapestry in understanding the matriarch's specialness. The doctor's mother soon becomes the reader's mother.

"The author's use of dialogue is often pure genius. To me the great conflict in the story, the guilt that Dr. Moss associates with negligence, runs so deep it disallows self-forgiveness. Dr. Moss can forgive, but will not accept forgiveness. Not only Shakespeare, it has Woody Allen written all over it.

"The prose is extremely literate, and some scenes are great literature. The autobiographical nature gives fundamental credibility to the son and his mother who are more than victims of a stroke — they are every mother and every son."

— John F.X. Ryan, Jr., Former Managing Director,
Sovran Limited and Pac West Distributing, Inc.
Executive Assistant, Lieutenant Governor,
State of Indiana

"I rate *Matilda's Triumph* a 10++! What a beautiful tribute to a mother's legacy. I appreciate the author's openness and willingness to share so much. I hope he experienced healing by sharing because there is no doubt that readers will be healed through this memoir.

"Matilda's strength of character as shown throughout will have her among the timeless matriarchs studied and compared in circles for years to come. What makes this book good is the context – stories of childhood, stories of Dr. Moss with his own children, and the story of his mother. But what make this book brilliant are the elements it contains that render it indispensable to literature as a whole.

"Matilda's struggles tightened her grip on the Jewish faith as the backbone to her legacy. She was unapologetic in her stand for Jewish devotion being noble and focused. It was her only constant other than the love of her children.

"Moss's complex, seemingly effortless ability to write – painting pictures with poetic language mixed with medical terminology is fascinating."

— Tiffany Moncrief
Editor of *Renew Partnerships*
Freelance Christian Writer

"I was swept into the story from the beginning. The tale was sweet, poignant, and heartwarming. At times, it was very heart wrenching and funny. The glimpse into the life of a colleague who I have known for years was both welcome and enlightening. The depth of feeling that was so apparent in his words and thoughts about his mother helped me to become immersed in the story. I shared many laughs and tears through the course of my reading. I would highly recommend this as a must read for anyone who has loved and lost."

— Lori Johnson, RN, Administrator,
Memorial Hospital Outpatient Surgery Center

"Dr. Richard Moss is a respected political and so-cial columnist in southwest Indiana. In his memoir, he turns the focus from the culture to his inner landscape and a description of his search for meaning in this very secular culture.

"Dr. Moss' search began with the needless murder of his teenage babysitter, his mother's critical illness, and the need to create or reclaim his own religious heri-tage. His journey becomes a struggle between inevita-ble fate and an emergent faith in the "God of Abraham, Isaac, and Jacob."

"His brother's fight with drug addiction and his mother's debilitating stroke both bring to a head a reli-gious crisis. In the end, he discovers that love is our in-evitable destiny, if life is to have any meaning. Through faith and grace, we can become more than just a narra-tive of our past."

— Rev. Deacon Thomas E. Holsworth, Ph.D., HSSP
Clinical Psychologist, Ph.D. from Purdue
M.S.T. St. Meinrad Seminary 2000

"This book will inspire people of all faiths and walks of life. Matilda, raising five boys in the Bronx proves to be entertaining; her amazing character shines through. She gracefully deals with all of the challenges life deals her. What a lady and what a story. You won't be able to put this book down."

— Nancy Blessinger
Registered Respiratory Therapist,
Christian mother

"Unlike highly touted and highly varnished auto-biographies of politicos who've done nothing, Rick's new book is an unvarnished bio of people who've done quite a lot, focused on two such: on Dr. Moss himself, a skilled surgeon who after years of pro bono volun-teering in Asia, established a conventional ENT practice in deepest Indiana; and on the life – soon following a major stroke – of his mother Matilda. She was an Indiana native, but a first-generation American born to a humble Sephardic family from the Balkans. The writing is fluid, compelling, informative and in the end genuinely uplifting and moving.

"Rick's childhood in the 1950s/1960s Bronx was nothing short of Dickensian, almost unimaginable to a taken-for-granted middle class reader like myself (also with solid Bronx and Brooklyn roots). There are semi-technical digressions on diagnostics, microbiology and pharmacology, and not least on medical ethics.

"Rick recounts his spiritual evolution from a six year old convinced he's born to be a prophet, literally, through the conventional irreligious radicalism of his university milieu, through a productive and respectful engagement with the Eastern traditions, and his continuing marriage to and professional partnership with Ying, a Sino-Thai nurse, who was rigorously converted into Judaism, but not necessarily out of Buddhism. Finally a philosophical re-engagement with Rabbinic Judaism – maybe Modern Orthodox Judaism."

— Alan Potkin, Ph.D., Team Leader
Digital Conservation Facility, Laos
Center for Southeastern Asian Studies
Northern Illinois University, De Kalb, IL.

"I was greatly blessed as I read this book. Richard Moss is transparent as he writes about his beloved mother and family. As a son, brother, husband, father and a trusting friend, he is an inspiration to many others and me. He is honest as he reports his mother's struggles to live. He explains his frustrations, hopes and guilt in the course of her illness. It is a story of faith, suffering, and redemption. I recommend it."

— Pastor Judith Branam, Jasper, Indiana
Apostolic United Pentecostal Church International

Matilda's
Triumph

Matilda's Triumph

A Memoir

Richard Moss, M.D.

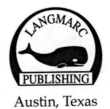

Austin, Texas

Matilda's Triumph
A Memoir
by Richard Moss, M.D.

Cover layout: Michael Qualben
Cover art © Wendel Field

Published by LangMarc Publishing
P.O. 90488
Austin, TX 78709
www.langmarc.com

Library of Congress Control Number: 2013948426
ISBN-10: 1-880292-86-6
ISBN-13: 978-1-880292-86-0

*I dedicate this book to my mother, Matilda,
a woman of passion, strength, and devotion.*

ACKNOWLEDGMENTS

The following friends and family members assisted me in the preparation and publication of this manuscript. John F.X. Ryan, Jr. was involved in this manuscript from the beginning, offering insights and encouragement. Scott Saalman and Richard Henson provided suggestions and careful editing that tightened and improved the story, as did Harvey Chaimowitz, who was ruthlessly honest in his criticisms. Nancy Blessinger saw in this account a chronicle of inspiration and triumph, suggesting a whole new approach to "pitching" it. Alan Potkin, Lori Johnson, Tiffany Moncrief, Judy Branam, and Tom Holsworth generously read and endorsed it. There have been others along the way, and I apologize for leaving any names out. Joe Schweiger provided photos of the Bronx. Wendel Field painted the canvas of my mother and the family tree (years ago), which became the book cover. Lois Qualben believed in the manuscript enough to publish it, for which I am grateful. She has devoted herself to the story and final product with energy and discernment.

I thank my wife for her patience, indulging my obsessions, and taking care of our four children while I huddled in the attic writing (and rewriting) the story. My four children, Arielle, Noah, Adina, and Isaiah, mean everything to me and the two oldest (Arielle and Noah) played vital roles in the story as they interacted lovingly with their beloved "Nona." Arielle's artistic photos on the Jewish star theme are inspired and appear in the book. My four brothers have encouraged me in the telling of our past. They reminded me of and provided background for many of the "Bronx" vignettes. My father was a colorful character who meant well. He struggled and gave us life. And then, of course, there was my mother . . .

FOREWORD

Matilda's Triumph is a memoirist's triumph. Part detective story, Moss, an otolaryngologist, becomes enmeshed in a medical mystery that takes him beyond the realm of his own discipline of expertise after his mother, who was visiting his southern Indiana home, suffers a debilitating stroke.

What follows is an honest, unflinching, personal account of the stroke's aftermath, its physical effects on Moss' mother, Matilda, and its mental effects on him. Moss becomes obsessed with finding all the information he can on strokes – its cause, its offal, its medicines. He is driven to restore his mother to a better quality of life – if she survives. When not tirelessly studying strokes, he prays – prayer and study, in essence, helping him escape the present.

While his mother remains unaware and in deep sleep for several days, Moss revives her, rebuilds her, via memories of his Bronx childhood in the '50s and '60s. His childhood accounts range from hair-raising to humorous to heartbreaking (his father left his family, leaving Matilda to fend for her five sons alone).

Other passages put Moss in the present, to reflections on his own wife, two children (at the time), his practice and his community (Jasper, Indiana). Moss must face the inevitability of his beloved mother's mortality, leaving the reader to witness a man caught between science and spirituality, guilt and forgiveness, as well as seeing him hit that hard brick wall of self-conceded helplessness, a hefty pill to swallow for capable physicians like Moss who are otherwise hotwired to be humble-free, hard-boiled and in hands-on control when facing their steady stream of patients whose lives become unbalanced due to difficult health issues.

Moss is a gifted, bona fide writer. There is not a lazy sentence left on the page. Each section is short, leaving the reader in want of more. *Matilda's Triumph* is a story of fathers, a story of sons, a story of mothers, a story of daughters, a story of brothers, a story of life, a story of death, a story of God, but ultimately, it is a love story – all neatly threaded into the fabric of a fantastic non-fiction read that left me at its end feeling exultant for having the good sense to read it.

Scott Saalman
Director, Employee Communications
Kimball International, Inc.
Jasper, Indiana

Prologue

Wealth and riches are in your home,
Your righteousness will
endure forever.
– Psalms 112

I didn't realize how far inside myself it all went, how deeply my mother had reached. She had always been there, and so I never saw life in any other way. From the moment of my birth, she had never been anything less than the soil I stood on and the air that sustained me.

But I had never taken its full measure, never understood its magic and complexity, the swarming tangle of roots and limbs that bound me to her. In some way, she still worked on me, the same as she had when I was a child. I still felt her presence, her memory lifting me as lightly as a leaf.

It was peculiar, perhaps, to talk this way at this age, as an adult, as a physician, but there was a frightening pain that came from such loss, no matter my years, a grief that welled up like a great wave that even the best of us could not resist.

My mother was ordinary in many ways, but by living a simple life and struggling with difficult circumstances, she taught vital lessons. I reflected often on this woman, my mother, who did not succumb.

She gave life to that which was incurable, where life had no right to take hold. She found meaning in never compromising, in clinging desperately to her truths, despite the tragedies, despite the misery, despite the uproar.

Richard Moss

As a memoir, this story maintains its veracity with respect to character, although some names and timing of events have been changed. Taken together, the narrative is a true account of a woman beset by inner demons, a son confronting his failures and guilt, and a family surviving in the inner city against harrowing odds. It is a chronicle of tragedy, duty, and the ultimate triumph of an embattled but determined mother.

-1-

Mom had left Indianapolis for New York as an eleven-year-old child with her eight siblings and parents in 1931, owing to a family scandal involving a divorce that by today's standards would scarcely raise an eyebrow. That meant that my four brothers and I would be raised in New York. It was a strange coincidence then, and not without irony, that I would grow up in New York City, only to return to Mom's home state of Indiana to live and build a medical practice.

September, 1998

It was the odd tilt to her head.

I was picking tomatoes in my garden with my son and daughter. It was early evening and the sun was low in the sky, producing that magical golden light that wrapped around you like a warm hand. Out of the corner of my eye, I saw my mother. She was visiting us for the month from New York City and had arrived last week, excited about being back in Indiana where she had grown up.

I noticed her walk out onto the patio in our backyard and immediately sit down on the lawn chair beneath the umbrella. It was not just sitting and relaxing though. There was something different. She almost seemed slumped over, her eyes closed, head tilted to the right. She had not acknowledged us, not even a wave of her hand or a nod.

1

"Mom, are you OK?" I called from a distance. There was no response, but she opened her eyes and looked my way. Maybe she didn't hear me, I thought and I returned to my children.

Her head still had that odd tilt, and she hadn't said a word or waved. Yet, three hours before, she had gotten into and out of my van without hesitation, not easy for a 78-year-old woman. We had gone to a local restaurant for lunch.

"Mom, are you OK?" I asked again as I walked toward her.

"Noahccccrrr wasshh cchhrr." Ungodly gibberish poured from her mouth, as if possessed. She was fighting with her dentures, unable to control her mouth or tongue.

"Mom, are you OK?" Could she be tired? Was she just waking up from a nap?

"Thaaatccchhh, Noahccchhhrr." The same slurred, demonic speech. Something about Noah, my three-year-old son.

"What happened, Mom?"

"Noahccchhr, that kid, I rrccchhhannnrr." Incomprehensible. About Noah again. "I ran up and downrrrcchhh." She had run up and down the stairs chasing Noah. But that wouldn't cause this. Her tongue seemed to hang, saliva pooled and trickled from the left corner of her mouth, and the left side of her face drooped. Her left arm and leg hung limply. Her right index finger kept tapping the metal armrest as if she were sending some kind of code.

"I was runncchhrr up andcchhrr down the stairscchhhhrrrr. I wasccchhhrrr worried about Noahc-chhrrrrr." By now, Arielle, my six-year-old daughter, and Noah had joined us. They heard Mom's weird gibberish, watched her struggling with her dentures, and heard the peculiar tapping of her right index finger on the armrest. At first, they laughed, thinking it was some kind of joke. Then they also realized that something was amiss. Arielle, especially, became worried.

"Nona, are you OK?" she asked.

"Yeah, honey, I'm tired," she said clearly. Thank God. Like flipping a switch. Maybe she was just tired.

"Are you OK, Mom?" I asked.

"Yeah, I'm OK."

Could Noah have just worn her out?

"What happened?"

"I donnnccchhh knowcccchhhh." There it was again.

"When did this start?" I asked.

"Rrggghhh." The same garbled speech and more tapping of her right index finger.

I wanted to see if it would just stop, but it didn't – it persisted, as obvious as a slap in the face - the mangled speech, the drooping face, the weird tapping of her right index finger. It was so abrupt and bizarre. Was she having some kind of psychotic break, some unexpected delusional leap after years of covert mental illness? Was she on medicines I did not know about?

Could it be a stroke?

A stroke? My mother was strong as an ox, could walk for miles. She had few risk factors. She did not smoke or have high blood pressure. She ate well. She had no history of vascular disease.

I had never seen a patient in the midst of an acute stroke. I had seen post-stroke patients with the slurred speech or hobbling around with a walker or consigned to a wheelchair – but never real time in progress. It was so unexpected. I struggled with the inconvenient facts. Cognitive dissonance, they called it: an unpleasant sensation that arose when one's experiences challenged one's beliefs. I looked at my mother. She was in trouble. Yes, my battleship of a mother, who had weathered a lifetime of storms, was in trouble.

As unlikely as it seemed, as unwanted as it was, I realized she was having a stroke. I picked up the phone.

"Brian, I've got a problem." I was talking to the ER doc on call at Memorial Hospital in Jasper, Indiana – a Chicago boy and a good physician.

"Yeah, Rick, what's up?" he said.

"It's my mother; I think she's had a stroke."

"What's she doin'?"

"She's slurring her speech and the left side of her face is drooping. I can't believe it. She's always been so healthy."

"It can happen, Rick. You have to bring her in."

"You can do something for her, I hope?" I asked.

"It depends. When did she have it?"

That was the question, wasn't it? At the time, I didn't think much about it.

"Just now, but I'm not sure."

"I'll talk to you when you get here. Does she have a doctor?"

"Regan."

The ambulance arrived at my home and the emergency medical technicians placed Mom on a stretcher, carried her into the back of the vehicle, and brought her to the emergency room. When we arrived, a nurse started an IV and sent her to have a CT scan. The emergency room doc called Bruce Regan, MD, an internist who already knew Mom. He came in and sized her up immediately: "She had a stroke, Rick. We'll have to admit her."

Everyone was sympathetic enough, yet it all seemed quite routine and casual. Not much you could do. How many thousands of these occurred every year?

"We'll start her on some heparin to thin her blood," Bruce said. "I'm sorry, Rick," he added, as he sat down to write some orders.

"Is there anything else we can do," I asked.

"It depends. TPA's an option. It's a potent anticoagulant. But Brian told me you weren't sure when the stroke started."

"I'm not certain."

"Were you with her before she had it?

"She walked out and sat down, and then she had the stroke."

"You weren't with her before she walked out."

"No."

"So, you don't know if she was having stroke symptoms before?"

"I don't know."

"When was the last time you saw her normal?"

"Three hours before."

"You have to be certain, Rick. TPA has to be given within three hours of the stroke."

"I'm not sure."

I sat with my mother in the emergency room. I was in a state of denial and depressed. Actually, I was in shock. I looked at her. The left side of her face still sagged and her left arm and leg were limp. It was strange to see her look at her left hand and attempt to move it, and fail utterly, as if a wire had been cut. The same with her left foot, right down to her toes. As hard as she tried, she could no longer summon these errant limbs to do her bidding.

"Mom, try to move your hand. Or just raise one of your fingers." Nothing. Zero. As in absolute zero, minus 423 degrees Kelvin, the temperature at which all movement, even little electrons careening about, ceased, frozen and crystallized into a rigid lattice; as in the deepest recesses of outer space, where the warming rays of the stars did not reach, and the temperature lifted not even a degree. Mom's hand was not cold, but its movement was frozen. An eerie stillness, it seemed, had descended upon her body, upon her left side.

I accompanied my mother in the elevator up to the third floor, the medical ward, where two nurses transferred her from the gurney to her hospital bed. They tucked her in, pulled the blankets, and adjusted the heparin drip.

"Are you comfortable, Mrs. Moss?" Mom sort of nodded. "We'll check on you later. If you need anything, just ring," one of them said, as if that should present no problem.

"Thanks," I said, and they left.

I sat down next to my mother, holding her hand. I explained to her what had happened and where she was, and she seemed to understand. Then she drifted off to sleep. I caressed her forehead and hand. I followed the methodical movement of her chest as she breathed. I watched the intravenous solution falling from the bag that hung over her bed and into the pump that regulated flow. The liquid, infused with heparin molecules, ran swiftly into her vein. To do what? God only knows, hopefully prevent any worsening of the stroke. It was soothing, though, to watch the fluid falling, drop-by-drop.

There was a distress light by the rail of her bed, a button to press if she needed something, placed properly on the right side, her functioning side. And a phone. Her small hands rested on her body. They were mirror images of one another, identical in appearance, yet quite different: the right one, alive and vital, touched still by essential life force, the other, limp and numb. Her face was wrinkled and tired, eyes closed. She slept deeply, as if nothing was wrong in the world, and yet what terrible event had occurred within her brain?

I gazed at my mother and wondered what lay ahead for this embattled woman. I thought about all that we had been through—she, my four brothers and me, back in the early days, in the Bronx, when my brothers and I were young and wild. We did not understand the torment my mother went through, the agonies she endured in raising us, and all that she had fought for in those hard but enchanted days, when she had watched over her brood like a lioness. I thought about the tragedies, the disappointments, and joys leading finally to this moment, with my once able and vigorous mother, now worn and withered, white haired and seventy-eight, cursed with a stroke, her left side useless, an invalid lying in a community hospital in the rural town of Jasper in southern Indiana.

My earliest memory of life was a night of thunder. I did not know if it was the thunder that crashed through the dark New York sky or the thunder that ripped across my forehead. And the daggers. The little daggers that played sharply upon my skull. It was a terrible night that nearly took me from the world before I had even started. I was two, and I recall nothing else before this.

I remembered wailing and thrashing, unable to form words, howling in pain. The pain throbbed and pounded inside my little head, and, finally, reached a crescendo that shook me like a leaf. I rose up inside my crib and grabbed the railing with chubby fingers, screaming, tears pouring from my eyes.

A door burst open, and three dark forms entered the room. A light switched on. It was my mother and two older brothers.

"Get me the knife," she said to one of them. She lifted me, "Oh, my boy, it's OK, Momma is here." She turned to the other brother. "Get me the alcohol and matches. Hurry!"

My brothers returned. My mother held me on her lap, wiping my forehead with the alcohol. She placed the blade of the knife into the alcohol, and lit it with a match. The knife blazed briefly like a torch and then quickly died out.

"Hold him down," she ordered. My two brothers put me on the floor and gripped me so that I could not move. My mother leaned down and held the knife over my infected forehead, swollen like a grapefruit.

"Don't let him move," she said, while I struggled to break free, bellowing like a ghost.

She positioned the knife at the center of the forehead where it seemed ready to burst, and, in one terrible stroke, jabbed the knife through the skin. They said I let out a horrible scream as green fluid shot out from the incision.

"Keep it out of his eyes," my mother yelled. My brother wiped the thick liquid, as my mother continued working the pus out through the opening.

"Gauze."

She poured alcohol onto the little pad and wiped my forehead.

"Tape," she said.

She taped the clean gauze pad in place over the incision and picked me up. The pounding and throbbing lessened. I was still screaming, but sensed, with my two-year-old mind, that the crisis had ended.

"That's a good boy," she said, stroking my head and kissing me.

"Is he alright, Ma?" one of my brothers asked.

"He's fine, son. It was just an abcess," she said calmly.

The two brothers sat on the floor next to my mother and in the dimly lit room, in the middle of the night, my mother sang sweetly:

> I love my Rick-a-la
> I love my Rick-a-la,
> I love you, I love you,
> I love Rick-a-la.

The pain had mercifully vanished. "Sleep, Rick, go to sleep," she said. The daggers and thunder had gone away, and I drifted off peacefully.

I don't know how my mother came to know what to do for she had no formal training. Perhaps it was something she had seen early in her life when people tended to illnesses at home and so felt able to manage it. I cannot say that this *event led me later to enter the world of medicine. I know only that she conveyed supreme confidence despite the urgency, and she greatly comforted me. I remember it to this day.*

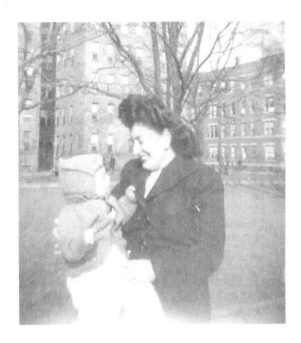

-2-

I stayed with my mother for several hours that first night, recollecting so many things about this mercurial woman who had raised me.

There were some qualities about my mother that had defined her, some peculiarities borne of necessity, of the anxiety of living too closely to the edge, without money and in dangerous places. Mainly, she was stubborn, in fact, one of the most stubborn and cantankerous persons I had ever known. But this did nothing to diminish my love for her. Because her stubbornness was nothing more than a survival mechanism, a normal, even healthy, reaction to an exasperating life. In fact, it was her greatest asset – raw, intractable mulishness that allowed her to endure.

She possessed another dominant quality – passion: a wellspring of fervor that matched her stubbornness. She did not direct her ardor at a glut of things, causes, or people, but a select few: the world of nature, her children, Judaism, Israel, and Harry, her husband, who left her forty years ago. Her passion was all consuming and easily ignited. It could manifest in a multitude of ways: intense anger, profound melancholy, ecstatic joy. The two forces at work within her, stubbornness and passion, were a formidable pair: the one rendering her immovable, the other amazingly volatile. Between them, she could be intensely protective. Or destructive.

But of all her passions, it was her children that engaged most of her vast energies, for it was her children who became her life's work, her one enduring creation. It was to this task that she threw herself and from which she extracted her greatest pleasure – and pain. She had other interests and talents, but none that approached this. When my father left her with five children many years ago for another woman, she subsumed all her other interests and passions to the single great task of raising us.

Of the five children, the five unmanageable boys that she gave birth to within a period of 13 years, there was one, in particular, whom everyone claimed received the lion's share of her devotion and affection. And that was her fourth son, me. Whether it was true or not was debatable, but the perception, at least, was there. Perhaps, in her heart of hearts, there was some seed of truth to it, for she never argued too arduously when my siblings raised the issue. The effect of that perception was profound.

I grew up with a sense of being the favored one, the chosen son, so to speak, of having, despite our humble origins, a sense of destiny – that same pesky sense of destiny that served only to complicate and disfigure one's life. Its effect on the others was a matter of conjecture. Did it flip a switch at some poorly lit depth within each of them resulting in a lowering of their own expectations, an early acquiescence in the great struggles of life – who knows? Whether I was truly her favorite in the first place was still an unresolved question, known only to my mother.

My mother used to say that she had five boys because she kept hoping to have a girl. After five failed attempts, she finally gave up. Other times, she claimed that she had so many kids because every time she and Dad fought, they had a baby. The story, though, could

not have been true, because Mom and Dad fought
much more than that.

I visited Mom early the next morning at the hospital
with my two children and was relieved to see that she
was alert and speaking more clearly. I asked her if she
understood what happened and she answered, "Yeah,
I had a sshhhtroke." Slurred but better. Although still
weak, her left side was regaining strength.

"Raise your left hand, Ma," I said. This time, the left
hand rose. Still weak, mind you, but movement just the
same. "Raise your left foot, Ma," and, again, it lifted.
"Wiggle your toes, Ma," and, lo, the toes wiggled. I
never before derived such unabashed pleasure at the
sight of functioning toes and fingers. It had a spiritual
or metaphysical dimension, a kind of resurrection, as
if the left side of her body had died and been miraculously reborn.

I was delighted, although my mother looked at me
oddly, perhaps wondering why the fuss over wiggled
toes. She was still a little confused, but no matter, for she
was on the mend. We sat with her for an hour, enjoying
ourselves, discussing the beautiful weather, making
plans for when she left the hospital. As we prepared to
depart, the children kissed their Nona and told her to
hurry home. Mom smiled at them and waved goodbye
with her right hand. I kissed her and left, feeling much
better than when I had walked in. Perhaps, it would
be only a small detour, and she could return home in a
few days.

Several hours later at work, in the afternoon, my
beeper went off. It was the hospital paging me. I called
back, concerned. I listened anxiously to the voice on
the phone: "Dr. Moss, your mother's taken a turn for
the worse."

"What is it?"

"She can't move her left side and her pulse is dropping."

"When did this start?"

"Twenty minutes ago."

"Did you call Dr. Regan?"

"Yes. He's coming in."

"What's her pulse?"

"About 45."

"Is she alert?"

"No."

"Can she raise her left hand?"

"No, not at all."

"What's her blood pressure?"

"90/60."

"What was it before?"

"120/70."

"What did Dr. Regan say?"

"He increased her IV fluids and ordered a CAT scan."

"She's getting heparin, right?"

"Yes."

"Did they do the CAT scan yet?"

"Yes, she's back now. We're taking her to the intensive care unit."

I ran to the hospital, up the stairs, and into her room. The nurses were with her, getting ready to transport her. I stood next to her and placed my hand on her forehead. I called out to her, "Momma," like a little boy. She did not respond. I became quite frantic, realizing how unprepared I was for this. "Momma," I said again, almost choking on my words. I spoke nervously to the nurses, barely able to complete my sentences.

"Is Dr. Regan coming in?"

"Yes, Dr. Moss, he's checking the CAT scan and will be right up."

"What's her pulse?"

"Still low."

"What is it?"

"40."

"And her blood pressure?"

"80/50." Damn, it's going down!

"Did he order anything?"

"No, but he's coming right up."

The nurses moved my mother out of the room. I watched as they wheeled the bed down the long corridor to the ICU. When I arrived, the nurses were busily attaching the probes that monitored her electrocardiogram and vital signs. I gazed at the luminous green panels above her bed that glittered and beeped.

"Momma," I called again, standing next to her.

"What are her vital signs?" I asked.

"Coming up, Dr. Moss," one of the nurses said. "Her heart rate is around 60 and her blood pressure's 100/70." *Thank God!*

I stayed with my mother, carefully watching her vital signs as they flashed across the screen. They were stabilizing. I did not know what happened, but, at least, she was improving. I watched her. She remained oblivious. I noticed my own vital signs stabilizing, too. I relaxed ever so slightly.

I had just survived a skirmish with something I now realized I was completely unready for: my mother's death. I felt as if I had evaded a catastrophe, yet, in reality, a reversal had occurred. But, death was the ultimate calamity, below which everything else seemed, at least, tolerable.

I had never seriously considered my mother's death. But when I watched her pulse drop, I suddenly found myself staring into the abyss. I became untethered, as if the various pieces of my mind had fragmented, and the center of my being had become lost. Perhaps, my relationship with my mother *was* the center of my life: this ancient, twisted snarl of memories, experiences, and emotions that formed the corpus of my tie with her, that linked me to her and, perhaps, all sons and mothers. With the prospect of its untimely end, I quickly devolved into a frightened orphan, shorn of the one essential bond that had sustained and defined my life. For the moment, at least, that process of disassembly had ceased, and I slowly gathered myself together again.

Relieved though I was to see my mother resting comfortably in her bed, the reality was that something terrible had happened, and the quick recovery I had envisioned earlier seemed now more distant.

Enfeebled, yes, I thought, as I sat down beside her, but how I recalled the enchantments she had sown.

It was a long time ago, but this is how I remember it ... When I was three, I took a walk with my mother through Crotona Park across the street from our apartment building in the Bronx. It was to my innocent eyes an immense park with hills, trees, and lakes, where children played all day and families ambled along dirt paths and wooded groves. It was spring, the sun was setting, and the sky was ablaze with bright fingers of orange and maroon. My mother was holding my hand as I looked at her. She closed her eyes and inhaled slowly, as if sampling the air like wine. She was beautiful to me, my mother, with full dark hair, warm eyes, and white skin, as pure as milk. She was my queen, and I her loyal subject, and joy for me was to be with her.

As the orange light reflected off her face, she paused, and looked at me with some urgency, saying, "Ricky, get me my paintbrush."

"Huh?" I said.

"... And my easel ... and canvas ..."

"Why, Mom?"

"And my paint."

"But why?"

"Because I want to paint."

"Paint what?"

"The sky!"

"Huh?

"I want to paint the sky!"

I looked at my mother. Could she do such a thing? I pictured her soaring, brush in hand, laying paint upon the heavens. Maybe she could!

"Ok, Ma, where do I get it?"

"I don't know, son, look."

I began scouring the area. I searched by a tree, around some flowers, in the grass. I checked under rocks, by a row of shrubs, near a bench. I found nothing. I looked at my mother. She smiled. Then she opened her arms, beckoning me. I was confused. Did she want the paint or not? I ran to her, and my Queen embraced me, showering my round face with kisses.

"Oh, you're a funny one, Ricky," she said, *"but that's OK, we'll just imagine we're painting the sky."*

"Why, Ma?"

"Don't worry," she said to her very earnest son, *"we'll paint it another day."*

And so I realized that my mother would not be communing with the heavens that day, at least not literally, not that I doubted she could. We continued our walk through the green meadows of Crotona Park, holding hands, content and at peace, capturing the final shafts of golden light as the sun drifted below the horizon.

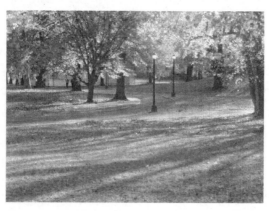

-3-

I spoke with Dr. Regan. He had seen her CAT scan and said that it was consistent with a large right sub cortical stroke. There was no evidence of hemorrhage, which, I supposed, was good, but her condition had worsened.

"Strokes are so unpredictable, Rick," he said sympathetically. "She was fully heparinized and it still progressed. You just can't predict them." He was frustrated.

Mom, Regan explained, had a variation in her circulation that predisposed her to this problem: the middle cerebral artery, usually gave off *several* vessels that supplied blood to the inner substance of the brain. These vessels were known as the *lenticulostriate* system. In Mom's case, however, the lenticulostriate vessels arose from a single trunk instead of multiple separate vessels.

When the stroke progressed, it involved not just a single perforating vessel but the entire system, cutting off circulation to a much larger region. The light stroke of yesterday in which Mom was still able to raise her left arm and leg progressed into a dense stroke with complete left-sided paralysis. The only redeeming feature of the calamity was that it involved the right side of the brain and not the left, thereby sparing her speech and cognitive centers.

This was no consolation. In fact, it was profoundly depressing. I now confronted the prospect of a protracted convalescence for my mother. As I contemplated the dismal facts, I remembered again the many trials she had endured in years past.

I was four. And my father was drunk.

"Why don't you ever come home at night," I heard my mother screaming in the kitchen.

My father was grinning and wobbling, enjoying a good drunk and the sight of his exasperated wife. He wore gray trousers, a white shirt with the collar open. She, a dress and apron. I opened the door of my bedroom where Jerry and I slept. We were afraid of the loud voices. I sensed a threat and possibility of violence.

"C'mon, Tilly, ya look beeyootiful," he said in his thick accent, as he reached for the hem of her dress, pulling it up. My mother cursed him and smacked him in the face.

"Get away from me, you!" she said angrily.

He never noticed.

"Ah, c'mon, Tilly, whuttsamatta witcha?"

"Get away from me!"

She threw a saltshaker at him. It hit him in the chest and burst open, spilling salt upon the floor. "And you stink. Don't come home drunk anymore."

Dad kept laughing. "Yaw beeyootiful when ya angry, Tilly. I mean it."

"Get outta my house."

"Whaddaya mean, yaw house?"

"Get out. And send me money. I've got five kids to feed, y'know."

Larry and Jack, the two oldest at 15 and 12, peeked into the kitchen. "Hey boys, come ova heah, look at how ya mudda's treatin' me." He was grinning and wobbling, occasionally coughing up huge clods of phlegm.

Larry and Jack entered the kitchen nervously. Larry, amazingly, stiffened and said, "Why don't you go, Dad?"

Dad underwent a rapid decompression. He turned to look at his first son, the one who dared to challenge him, and casually lit a cigarette. After a moment, while taking a drag, he said, "Yoo tawkin' to ya fadda like dat?"

"It's just better," Larry answered.

"Who tawt ya ta tawk like dat," he said, a tinge of menace in his voice.

"No one, Dad. It would be better if you just left, that's all."

"Ya still openin' ya big yap ta me?"

"Yeah, Dad," he said, determined.

And Dad rose up on his heels, full of a father's rage for the disobedience of his son. "Where do yoo getoff tawkin' like dat, ya nogood punk?" he said, raising his right arm about to backhand Larry across the face when suddenly Mom ran and pushed him from behind, sending him sprawling against the sink and onto the floor.

"Get outta here, you sonofabitch," she screamed, "get outta our house!"

Dad went berserk. He picked up the chairs and smashed them. He hurled dishes and cups. He splintered the table and emptied the cabinets. He cursed and raged, a vortex of destruction that left the kitchen in ruin. Mom stood in the middle of the chaos and glared at him. Dad, for his part, never laid a hand on her. When the dust and fury had settled he said, "I'm neva' comin' back."

And he was gone. We stood there amidst the carnage in silence.

It was the late fifties, before the excesses of the latter part of the next decade, the sixties and beyond, had been felt. Broken homes had not yet come to litter the landscape as commonplaces. The drug scene that would consume the neighborhood in the coming years had not yet exploded onto the streets as they would, making only cameo appearances here and there on street corners or parks at night.

Blacks and Puerto Ricans were moving in, altering the flavor and texture of the area, and Spanish could be heard in the streets. It was still a "Jewish" neighborhood, but changing quickly, both demographically and culturally. The Bronx was relatively safe, but it would not stay as such. And we began to hear more about robberies, hold ups, and shootings occurring within our midst.

We lived on a tree-lined street next to a city park, Crotona Park, with trails, a lake, and small forested areas, not an unpleaant place at all, considering the urban colossus that surrounded it. But here, too, Mom always cautioned us about the neighborhood and refused to let us walk in the park at night.

There were other apartment buildings on our street, some private homes further up, then a junior high school, PS 44. Shecters was a small grocery store on the corner and the "El" on Boston Road and 174th, a busy street with supermarkets, pizzerias, and a movie theater, were just blocks away.

In the living room we had a 13-inch black and white TV and a "hi-fi." My mother listened to George Gershwin and Nat King Cole on vinyl records.

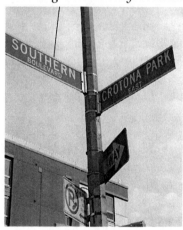

Six unhappy souls, my mother and her five boys, were left alone in our cramped two-bedroom apartment with chipped paint and cracked walls, a five-story walk-up on Crotona Park North. Each of us would feel the impact of Dad's stormy departure in the weave of our troubled family and upon us individually.

-4-

I contemplated the anomaly of my mother's cerebral circulation. It was an accident of fate but one that had contributed to a significant event – the transformation of a minor stroke to a major one with complete hemi-paralysis. It was not the only factor but an important one. And it was something she had no control over. She was born with it, just as she was born with brown hair and light complexion. Only now, seventy-eight years later, it revealed itself, a bit of bad luck.

She had an ischemic stroke, not a hemorrhagic one, which meant that a vessel had not ruptured and bled into the tissues, but rather that a thrombus had formed and shut off blood supply. A thrombus. This was a muscular medical word, almost onomatopoetic. A thrombus was a clot, an accumulation of vascular debris that plugged a blood vessel.

In the "original" plan, before people lived so long and died young of causes other than heart disease and stroke, the ability to clot or form a thrombus was desirable; and still was – in other contexts. Clotting allowed injured vessels to seal themselves and kept us from hemorrhaging to death when we cut ourselves, a thoroughly life-sustaining physiology. Clotting, or thrombus formation, though, in settings other than that of a severed or ruptured vessel was undesirable. It reflected a breakdown or disruption in the complex mechanisms that maintained the normal flow and fluidity of blood.

21

In modern days, with people no longer dying of small pox, temperature extremes, or malnutrition, individuals enjoyed the privilege of living longer and dying of other causes, most commonly *thrombogenic* (clot forming) vascular disease, the contemporary equivalent of the bubonic plague. Was it that bad? Of course. Millions upon millions died each year from strokes and heart disease.

So my mother had had a thrombus that plugged a vessel that fed a particular area in the brain that contained nerve tracts that traveled down the spinal cord and made possible purposeful body movement. A micro-event with devastating effects.

With the unhappy circumstance of my mother's stroke, I realized how ignorant I was of its pathophysiology. Shame for a doctor, however specialized, even as an otolaryngologist.

How did strokes begin? What were the causal factors? How to prevent and treat them? I began to study the subject, delving into the tiresome texts, immersing myself in the esoterica and minutiae. I felt obliged, a personal and even religious responsibility.

Jewish tradition had always encouraged study, emphasized its sacred nature, of the scriptures and law, yes, but of secular subjects as well, particularly the healing arts. I reviewed articles, scoured the literature, and talked with colleagues. I realized quickly what a complex and intensely studied area it was. Not that I was surprised, for cerebrovascular disease, *stroke*, was no small matter. It was, in fact, Leviathan, an appalling behemoth that, eventually, either personally or through loved ones, affected everyone.

I was in my study, closing one such voluminous text on the subject when I heard a knock on the door. I turned to find Arielle standing before me. I smiled at her, surprised.

"Daddy, what happened to Nona?" she asked. I admired the clarity of her question. What, indeed, *had* happened? She did not seem troubled, only inquisitive. She was also adorable and I could not resist her. I gathered her up and kissed her.

"That, my little flower, is a good question." I placed the volume on the shelf and looked at her. "Nona had a stroke," I began.

"What's that, Daddy?"

"It's something bad that happens in someone's brain."

She appeared no more enlightened. I thought better how to explain it.

"Do you know what happens when you cut yourself?" I said, taking a different tact.

"Uh huh."

"What happens?"

"You bleed."

"Right. How does the blood get there?"

She shrugged.

"Blood vessels," I said.

"What's that?"

"Those are little tubes that carry blood all over the body. Blood is important because it brings food and oxygen to the body." I could see I was losing her. "You know, when you eat food, the vitamins and minerals in the food are absorbed by the blood and carried all over the body to make you strong. And the air you breathe through your lungs when you take a breath." I inhaled deeply to make the point. Then she took a breath. "See. Air has oxygen. You're breathing in oxygen because your body needs it. And you eat because you're body needs food."

"Uh huh."

"These little tubes or 'vessels,' we call them, *blood vessels*, carry blood with all the good things – the food and oxygen – around the body." I looked at her, making sure she was still with me.

"Uh huh," she nodded.

"In older people, sometimes blood vessels get clogged."

She nodded.

"A stroke happens when a blood vessel in the brain gets clogged. Part of the brain will starve because without blood it has no food or oxygen. And the brain is the busiest part of the body, because it has to think and watch over everything else."

"Uh huh."

"And then the brain can't take care of the body. That's what happened to Nona. One of those little blood vessels in her brain clogged up and part of the brain stopped working. That's why she can't move. A stroke is like a plug in a blood vessel, or maybe we can call it a crumb, because that's all it takes to block the vessel - a little crumb."

"Will Nona be OK, Daddy?"

"I hope so, honey."

Satisfied, she ran off.

I felt I had engaged in the highest form of exegesis. Better yet, she seemed to understand.

Jason Braun, MD, the neurologist, stopped by my office unexpectedly the next morning.

"Hi, Jason, how are you?"

"Hello, Rick. Can I speak with you," he asked.

"Sure," I said, and we entered my private office.

"I'm so sorry, Rick."

"Yeah, out of the blue."

"She was just coming for a visit?"

"Yes."

He looked at me sympathetically. "She's never had problems before?"

"No," I said.

"No risk factors? Regan mentioned her cholesterol was a little high."

"Age, weight, mild diabetes. She was strong as an ox."

"Anything else?" he asked.

"She had surgery for lung cancer four years ago but sailed through it. Been disease free since."

"I wish you had called me about this," he said.

I looked at him.

"It could have made a difference."

I nodded slowly.

"We could have started her on TPA."

"I-I spoke to them about that in the ER," I said. "I wasn't sure when the stroke began. I thought it had to be within three hours."

"I'd have started her on it, anyway."

"She was fully heparinized when the stroke progressed," I said.

"The TPA is far more potent; it might have dissolved it."

"There are risks with TPA," I said.

I finished out my day in the office, but something had happened, as if I had blown a fuse somewhere. The conversation with Jason haunted me. I labored through the day, my own words agitating me. I knew about TPA, how effective it was with heart attacks, but did not realize its usefulness for strokes. There were issues of timing and risks associated with it. But that mattered little now with my mother's left side useless. Where was I when the moment of decision arose, when I brought her to the ER?

I confronted now fresh deposits of guilt, a noxious presence that coiled inside me. One thought dominated all others: I had failed my mother. A single pivotal moment to act missed, followed quickly, like many such events, by a rapid descent into chaos.

"How is your mother, Rick," my wife Ying, asked that evening when I returned home. Ying was Thai, of Chinese ancestry, a nurse I met while traveling and working in Asia as a surgeon years ago.

"Stable, that's about it."

"I will visit her tomorrow," she said.

Ying had never forgiven my mother for the cool reception she had given her when we returned from Asia in 1990. We had to stay with Mom in her small apartment in New York City to save money. It was not comfortable, and Mom did not welcome her newest daughter-in-law. Mom resented all five of her daughters-in-law. Ying was just the latest in a string of female usurpers who had assumed the central role in the lives of her sons.

"She's not moving her left side at all?" she asked.

"No, she barely responds."

"She can still recover," Ying said.

"How do you know?"

"I took care of stroke patients in Thailand," she said.

"You did?"

"Yes."

"You've seen them get better?"

"Some of them - yes."

I felt something ease up in me.

"Jason Braun, the neurologist, stopped by," I said.

"What did he say," she asked.

"That I should have called him."

"Why?"

"He would have given her TPA."

"What's that?"

"A blood thinner, used for heart attacks – and for strokes, too."

"So you're blaming yourself?"

"Yes."

"It wasn't your fault," she said sympathetically.

I had no choice now. I had to study. I needed it to stop the noise and the sense of utter buffoonery that consumed me. The TPA thing was now a recurring theme that I could not shut off. My thoughts ran to it, like a tongue to an open sore. The weight of my failure oppressed me. And study, which compelled me to understand my mother's illness, aggravated my sudden neurosis. Was there anything else I could have done?

I opened the text again, alone in my room. I glanced at the dark grain of my mahogany desk. I leaned back in my swivel chair. I dimmed the overhead light as the ceiling fan spun, creating soft eddies of air that swept around me. I would be OK, I told myself. A fly buzzed annoyingly around my head as I thumbed the pages. It was a weighty volume, possessed of much *gravitas*, a typical medical book. I read a fragment here and there, dry and unimaginatively written, yet for me engaging, filled with morsels that I devoured in ghoulish fashion.

It was more than a religious duty now, well beyond that, if such a thing could be said, for I was drawing close to the underside of my being, a morass of disconnected sensations and images, a noxious cloud of random memories and thoughts that coalesced around the base of my brain like a tumor. I could not ask God for help. I had to arrange myself in more tidy fashion before petitioning Him, the Lord of the Universe. It was a sordid thing now, more a question of survival, for I felt myself threatened. The invisible fibers that harnessed my being were unraveling before the acid of self-loathing.

I read on. Line upon line, page upon page, table upon table, graph upon graph, the endless trail of data and conjecture, the substance of medicine, the monotonous chronicle of death and disease. I must secure myself before anything else; undo the cycle of contempt that had metastasized within me. In the aftermath of my failure to act, I became driven not just by the desire

to understand her disease, but by an ambition to restore her - and in so doing, of necessity, restore myself,
for I felt my bloodless self slipping into obscure realms.
    I continued to read.

Plaque was the protagonist in the opening scene in the story of
stroke, for here was its genesis, the name given the lesion lodged
within the wall of an artery from which so much misery and unhappiness emerged. It was the offending lesion associated with the disease process known as atherosclerosis: an atherosclerotic plaque,
as opposed to a dental plaque or a psoriatic plaque. For these others were wholly pedestrian affairs, mundane and trivial, unlike the
redoubtable atherosclerotic plaque that so transfixed me.

But plaque was where the evil process began, an unwanted
slick of oil within the arterial wall, just within the inner lining, the
endothelium. It was here where the damage began, for as the fatty
deposit grew, it deformed the vessel and narrowed its passage, finally disrupting the inner lining, bursting into the bloodstream itself,
its grotesque and twisted form now washing up against the rushing
tide of blood and all the tiny life elements swirling about - including
platelets, those minuscule creatures - mere cell fragments - that
contained the necessary biochemical machinery that brought the
great drama to its logical end.

Platelets transformed themselves, became sticky, attracted
others, and filled the stricken vessel. They were the confused
agents of death, the unwitting foot soldiers of doom, and they fed
upon the plaque by the thousands, by the millions, attracted to it
like bright flies.

I woke up early the next morning, while it was still
dark, rolling about miserably. It was three days since
the stroke. The kids were in bed next to me, sleeping
soundly; they had slipped in last night under cover of
darkness. I did not want to wake them. Ying, I noticed,
was not in bed. Did she suffer from insomnia as well? I
put on my bathrobe and went down to the kitchen. She
was there, drinking coffee.

"You did not cause the stroke," she said.

"I know that."

"The medicine may not have helped her."

"Maybe, we don't know."

"She can still recover."

I went to see Mom in the Intensive Care Unit (ICU) that morning, before going to my office. I felt the same sense of gloom and anxiety that began after my conversation with Braun. I could not shake the weight of my guilt, my profound sense of failure. And I could barely contain an inexplicable unease I felt as I walked towards the hospital. I steeled myself for the unpleasantness as I approached the building.

It was a curious path to the ICU, positioned as it was in the back of the building away from the front entrance. Then it was the long hike to the back elevator.

I passed the friendly middle-aged women with the headsets at the admission booths and then radiology. I hurried by the pharmacy representative table where an appealing, smartly dressed female drug "rep" recited the virtues of the particular snake oil she was peddling. I did not smile, social niceties well past my powers now. I strolled past the laundry department with the immense industrial washing machines, cleaning the linens and garments of the sick, the dying, and the dead, past the pathology department – the FBI of the hospital. This is where all the biopsies and resected body parts were sent to be pickled, sliced, and analyzed, beside the microbiology lab where bodily fluid specimens (blood, urine, sputum) found their way to be examined or cultured.

Then came the pastoral office where the kindly *sister*, a nun in civvies, prepared for her morning rounds. I turned a corner and came upon a small recess in a hospital cul de sac with a rarely used elevator. I rode to the third floor, marched alongside the neonatal unit, behind the happy faces ogling their newest relative through a glass window, to the ICU waiting room and into the ICU.

Mom was still asleep when I entered the room, amidst the beeping noises and monitors. I adjusted myself again to her unhappy reality, my mother floating senselessly in a mirage of sounds and lights that meant nothing, offering only an unintelligible language that scraped against some rough surface within myself, an abrasive and caustic texture. There was an undercurrent of apprehension in this room, a foreboding that resonated between the weird sounds and disturbing echoes, as I stepped to her bed. Was it something imagined or simply invisible?

I watched the droplets of fluid fall from the IV bag, still crammed with the heparin that had not helped her, running swiftly through the tubing and into her vein. It induced a state of meditation, captured my attention, and registered as something soothing. Were the falling drops of fluid the analog of my heart? Were the two in harmony with one another? There were EKG probes on her chest depicting her cardiac rhythms, forming eerie green tracings on the monitor. A pulse oxymeter attached to her index finger, gently grasping the digit, counting red corpuscles as they streamed through her capillaries, configuring its tally as numerical figures on a screen. I felt the weight again of my senses and the unwanted visions.

"Momma," I spoke, and for one brief moment, she stirred. She opened her eyes and then drifted back to sleep. "Momma," I called out again, but this time there was no answer. She had returned to the silent spaces within. What was the process at work here? Why the profound slumber? Was it better for her to slip between the folds of her mind and remain incognito?

The nurse walked in. "Hello, Dr. Moss." She smiled. "She is doing OK," she said, "vital signs are stable." She wore a navy blue nursing uniform, was middle-aged and slightly over weight but had a pleasing expression. She grasped my mother's hand. I liked the nurse's face, positioned as it was between stages of life, matronly but still attractive, a welcome sparkle present in her pupils; she wore cherry red lipstick, still possessed, as she was, of womanly spirits.

After a point, the animal passions eroded, like so much dross, replaced instead with a dull buzz echoing between the ears and a stuporous glaze to cover it all. It was, I supposed, inevitable, the arthritic process at work upon ourselves, the gradual accumulation of life's ceaseless banalities yellowing our vision.

"Does she respond at all?" I asked.

"No, not really, but I don't try too hard to wake her either."

It was not, after all, a small injury she suffered, a flesh wound or sprain, but something much deeper, something that ran to the very core of things. All we saw was the body with eyes closed. Not a coma and not death either, although there were disturbing similarities.

"Her respiratory rate is good, heart rate and blood pressure's been fine," she said.

Was she reading my mind? For at that very moment I was watching Mom's chest, assuring myself that she was, indeed, still breathing, carefully observing the subtle rising and falling of her chest in gentle cadences. So silent and fixed was she, that despite the green squiggles upon the monitor above her bed, I needed a more visceral form of evidence.

"So she seems stable," I said.

"Yes."

A stroke was a different sort of beast really, not amenable to quick fixes. I could not talk my way out of this, not plead, beg, or borrow. I was powerless, and she was asleep. I could only wait, nothing more. The moment of judgment had passed and left me with the aftermath of my indecision.

"How long before I can take her home?" I asked, almost facetiously.

"I don't know," she answered, not getting my sarcasm; for I knew it would not be soon.

I requested a stethoscope. I wanted to hear my mother's heart, experience the aging muscle still throbbing within her chest as it received and expelled blood, the very heart that had labored for both of us when I was percolating along within her womb more than forty years before. The sounds were all there, as I knew them, the familiar thrashing of that small fist, plodding tirelessly, as dim and monotonous as could be, but the *glory* of those wondrous chambers and valves pounding into eternity!

I navigated around her chest, listening gratefully to the deep emissions of air entering and leaving her lungs. The joyous sounds invoked calm, a further confirmation of her fundamental intactness. The essential organs were still busily at work within her, striving admirably under the circumstances, and keeping her, thank God, fastened to the earth, even as her brain and mind had temporarily skipped off to mend themselves.

Her heart and lungs worked in tandem, perfectly timed, and complementing one another, woven into a perfect dance that sustained life, a daily and parochial event, but a miracle, nonetheless! Her breath sounds were cavernous, the radioactive air sweeping in from some far-flung corner, carrying its electric force. It alighted within her, releasing its essence, and then blew out to mix with the elements. Yet, for a single instant, that volume of breath was as intimate with my mother as could be. I handed the stethoscope back to the nurse, strangely relieved.

"Her oxygen saturations are good, pressure's holding, and her heart rate's OK," the nurse offered.

"Good," I answered. But the deeper questions remained. "Why is she so sleepy?"

"It's typical," the nurse answered, not unkindly.

"Her synapses and nerve transmission are slow," I murmured, more to myself. This much I had unearthed already in my forays into the neurological sciences.

"It'll take time, Dr. Moss. The ones we get in are usually somnolent for three or four days." This, the subtle, probably unintended reminder of how routine these disasters were. She meant to reassure me.

"She needs the rest," the nurse said.

"Right."

She felt her pulse, as an after thought.

And I sat with my mother who slept in the silent spaces, communing in the darkness from which no light emerged. And I remembered other trials.

When my father stopped coming around, I always wondered where he went and whether he had another house. How could you have two houses? There was only one home, one house, I thought. Did he live in the street or stay with his mother and father, like he did when he was a kid? I met his Mom and Dad a couple of times, and I remembered his father was bald, except for some white hair on the sides, and heavy. He wore suspenders, smoked cigars, and had a funny accent. He was from Russia, Mom had told us. We never saw much of him. My brother Jack told me that Dad was a barber and he worked in his dad's barber shop, an old time place with the spinning barber pole outside. He went to high school but not college.

After Mom kicked Dad out of the house, she worried a lot. She worried about how to take care of the kids and how to pay for everything we needed. The five of us had to eat, not to mention have clothes and books. There was the rent, the telephone, and electricity, and so many things that she could not afford. She asked Uncle Willy, her brother, who was Dad's good friend, if he knew where Dad was, but he had not seen him. One of Mom's friends told her to call the police on him for child support, but she would not.

"I can't call the police on the father of my kids!" I heard her say on the phone. Somebody told her to go to the relief office, but Mom refused. "Go on relief?" she said. "I would rather starve then go on relief."

Mom, who had a high school education, supported us by working downtown as a receptionist in the "garment district," then centered in downtown Manhattan. These were the days when clothing was actually made in the United States, and New York City was the garment capital of the world. Every morning Mom arose early, got us off to school, and walked to the train on Boston Road and 174th Street. She rode down into the bowels of the city to 42nd Street where she worked. She returned after five, the same hour ride back, shopped, carried the groceries, and cooked for her five boys.

At night, we sat around the little table that Mom bought after we threw out the one Dad smashed, with the old chairs Mom found in the back yard that someone threw out. We were eating spaghetti and each of us had a half cup of soda, except Larry and Jack, because they were older, had a full cup. We had pineapple slices for dessert. After dinner, Jerry and Jack cleaned off the table. Mom began washing the dishes. She turned the faucet on. She put soap on the sponge. She checked the water to make sure it was hot and told us to bring the dishes over to her. Someone had to clean the stove. Someone had to dry the dishes and put them on the shelf. Someone had to sweep under the table and around the kitchen and put the leftovers away. Someone had to take out the garbage.

Each night, while washing the dishes, Mom would sing a familiar song, singing to herself as if she were alone in her own world. She began by humming the melody, and then she would sing it, a sad song with a sad sound. I didn't know it was a famous song at the time; I thought it was her own song. She sang:

"Somebody loves me,
I wonder who,
I wonder who he can be ...
Somebody loves me
I wish I knew,
Who can he be worries me ...
Somebody loves me,
I wonder who,
Maybe it's ..."

("Somebody Loves Me"
by George Gershwin)

And she never finished the last line. She closed her eyes, still wearing her work clothes and high heels and lipstick, washing the dishes. She sang this song as if she were dreaming about someone, maybe Dad, wishing he'd return and be her husband again, happy with his five kids, raising them like families were supposed to, instead of alone with no one to help and no money, struggling all the time. Tears would form and roll down her cheeks and into the dirty dishwater, onto the dishes and cups and sponge.

She kept cleaning as she cried, repeating this refrain, unable to finish that line, mixing her tears with the dishwater, as if blessing it. The brothers were busy, except Cliff who was still too young, but we all knew she was crying. We knew the familiar sounds. When she finished, she opened her eyes as if coming out of a dream. She looked around the cramped kitchen with the chipped paint, the ripped linoleum, and the five boys who depended on her for everything.

-5-

I left my mother in the ICU as I found her, asleep.
I ran to my office. It was a busy day, the schedule full.
The complaints of my patients, the aches and pains,
the symptoms drew my professional attention but I
was preoccupied. Private practice was often a litany
of minor affairs, punctuated by an occasional authen-
tic medical crisis that galvanized and inspired. It could
sometimes be tedious, a spectrum of elective maladies
that required a fraction of one's total medical skill. Still,
it was an important service in our small community.

But it was the opposite of my experiences in Asia in
which I encountered horrendous misfortune routinely.
I cut my teeth there, but ran out of money, and so could
not continue my Great Adventure, the grand contest
that pitted me against the grotesqueries of my voca-
tion, the massive and disfiguring cancers of the head
and neck that abounded in that vast continent. It was
noble and compelling, and I always hearkened back to
those days.

To a certain extent, I lived my life in the past, as
if I had already seen my best and most heroic years.
I wanted to return to my work overseas, but for now,
there was only this, my practice, my children, and pres-
ently my stricken mother, to whose downfall I had contributed. I managed to complete my day without making a fool of myself. Afterwards, I went to the office of
Jason Braun, MD. It was four days post stroke.

"Is Dr. Braun free?" I asked the receptionist.

I knew that Jason was off on Wednesday afternoons and often did paperwork at that time.

"I'll see if he's available, please have a seat." I picked up a magazine. The waiting room was empty. It was tastefully decorated and no kiddy play things like I had in my office for my pediatric patients. There were several impressionist paintings on the walls and an abstract sculpture with a polished, rounded surface, quite soothing to the eye.

There was a table in the center of the room, a rack with magazines, and, thankfully, no TV. I noticed the framed photo of him playing a clarinet on one of the walls, and I remembered he was a musician. It was a pleasant room with a bland but calming atmosphere. The receptionist reappeared. "He can see you now." She led me to his room. He was already standing, ready to greet me.

"Rick, how are you?" he said as I entered.

"Fine, thanks," I said, sitting down in front of his desk.

"I'd have taken a chance and given her the TPA, Rick," he said, cutting quickly to the point. "Even if you weren't sure of the exact onset of symptoms. I have seen dramatic turn-arounds. Yes, you are right, there are risks, but it's a risk worth taking."

"What are those risks?"

"Hemorrhage. From leaky capillaries. It has to be given within three hours, or else they can bleed," he said.

"But I have seen patients walk out of here after bad strokes using TPA. I have seen strokes vanish. The clots disappear. I have saved brains with TPA," he said emphatically.

"But what about the onset of symptoms," I said. "It has to be within three hours of the stroke. It's not like a heart attack, where you have all day. The heart and the brain are different things, different tissues. One's a big muscle. The other's a bag of fat and water."

"You're right," he said. "But I think you were within the time constraints. Maybe, you weren't sure, but I think, from what I heard, you were within the three-hour limit."

"How do you know?" And I thought angrily to myself, why hadn't I tried to determine the exact time frames.

"Probability, that's all. I'd have nailed the time issue down, gotten as close as we could to knowing when it started, and then we'd have discussed probability and risk. And it'd have been up to you."

With this, he pushed the dagger in fully.

"Alright," I said despondently, "tell me about TPA."

"Tissue Plasminogen Activase. It is a thrombolytic agent. The initial work was with MI's. Stroke is relatively recent. The landmark study was NINDS." (MI's are myocardial infarctions or heart attacks)

"NINDS?"

"Yes, the National Institute of Neurologic Disorders and Stroke study."

"What about it?"

"TPA is the ultimate clot buster. Great with hearts and helpful with strokes, but it has to be given within three hours – that's the drawback. Longer than that and the risk of bleeding is too high. I have used it often. It is a miracle drug – but there are limits."

"So what do we do now?"

He shrugged. "I will evaluate her. We can anticoagulate her and begin the usual things, rehab, therapy, and the like."

"There's nothing else, some agent to enhance recovery, neuroprotective agents, nutrition, anything?" I asked.

"We'll, perhaps, there are research protocols. I will see what is available. But please understand, Rick, it was a dense stroke."

When I returned home, dinner awaited me. I ate with disinterest. The kids were upstairs watching TV. I usually limited their TV watching. I preferred they sit with me during dinner, followed, generally, with some light activity afterwards – a walk, a catch, a bike ride. Now it seemed easier to let them follow their own inclinations, which inevitably led them to the courtyard of the television. Perhaps, it would have been wiser to have them join me for dinner with some pleasant diversion to follow, culminating in their bedtime story and sleep.

This was our pattern now, established over six years, and it worked well. I had climbed fully into the role of father, a spontaneous transformation that occurred the moment I first spied my daughter squirming from her mother's womb, pink and writhing, covered with a cheesy layer, howling from the shock of life, her little eyes blinking in wonder. Then once more with her little brother, Noah – the same process, differing only in details. The successive stages of growth and development, as they passed through them, enhanced the bond that began at their births.

It had nothing to do with sentimentality or even emotions. Rather, it derived from some subterranean fixation, beneath conscious awareness, engraved in the hook-up of neurons, or, perhaps, even more sublimely, on the order of biochemical structure and flow, the arrangement of nucleotides, the genetic code. It took care of itself, needed no prompting or instructions, certainly no parental guidebooks, seminars, magazine articles, or whatever rigmarole someone had cooked up in this frivolous little culture of ours.

But I took the night off from all that, left the children to their own devices and followed mine. I abandoned my wife at the table and returned to my study. I switched the light on and surveyed the books on the dark wooden shelves.

I plunged once more into the area of my dilemma. Today it was thrombogenesis (again) or "clotting," a dismal (but central) process, a continuation of yesterday's review.

Thrombogenesis was a bewildering affair, amazingly ticklish, and always teetering on disaster, based, as it was, on a dizzying multitude of factors, enzymes, and reactions, all of which had to be maintained in precise balance for things to proceed properly. That tragedy did not occur more often than it did was a vivid testimonial of the underlying genius of it all. The mechanism, though, whether as part of the atherosclerotic process leading to a stroke or as part of the coagulation pathway that prevented bleeding, ran quite parallel. In fact, they were identical. It was, in brief, a complex cascade of reactions that activated platelets. And platelets became the primary player in the coagulation scheme.

The critical issue was that platelets lacked the capacity to distinguish between a vessel injured by an animal bite, a scrape, or the tip of a spear, say, and the same vessel injured by a ruptured plaque. Programmed through eons of evolutionary tinkering, platelets bound tenaciously to damaged vessels for whatever reason. They did not know better. The primary purpose of the platelet was to seal rents in vessels, regardless of the cause. This feature of the platelet developed through epochs when people (and animals) lived short and brutal lives, generally enhanced survivability as it did today. Now, though, we lived longer and developed vascular disease, and the blind hemostatic urge of platelets in the setting of atherosclerosis worked unhappily against us.

I closed the book.

It was unintentional. The platelets were tools in the larger scheme, careless cellular automatons. Incapable of conscious thought, they were, of course, blameless. Morality and virtue were realms apart from their tiny worlds. Should I continue the study of the mechanics of stroke, devoid of moral imperative, immersed in the play of science, as a child dabbling in a candy store?

It was cool to the touch, science was, as it should be: dispassionate, understated, not biased or polemical, not given to exaggeration or rhetoric (unless, of course, taken hostage for political purposes). It did not sear or singe, nor did it console or make promises. It did not pursue agendas or promote consensus. That was not its purpose. It only dissected and analyzed small fragments in highly controlled settings, to provide bits of data, moving the scientific endeavor forward in miniscule increments; it sought only valid, reproducible outcomes, not contrived or manufactured ones, bringing us closer to some corner of the truth, regardless, mind you, of "consensus." It could never answer broad or ultimate questions, say, the origin of life, the nature of consciousness, or even the variation of species, for that matter, notwithstanding the howling of the Darwinists who worshipped at the altar of scientific materialism.

But it served its purpose now – distracting me, passing the time, and somehow serving as a kind of compress, perhaps by creating the illusion that I was actually doing something to heal my mother.

Ying entered the study. It was time for the children to go to bed, and bedtime stories, whatever the contingencies, were indispensable. "They're waiting upstairs for Daddy," she said. Somehow, this flicker of normalcy was utterly comforting, the reprieve of bourgeois life. Perhaps, my children would repair me.

I could lapse into an ever-deepening funk, a repetitive internal denigration that lead me only further into darkness and the loss of structure. Madness and despair beckoned. I could tabulate the sequence, and measure the steps that led me there, envision the process, which in itself was frightening. And the self-correcting mechanisms may not withstand the assault, could abort themselves, or be overcome by the counter-vailing forces.

I had had these tendencies before, but somewhere from within, had always resisted that movement, navigated carefully through the labyrinth to some berth of light and air. But just being aware of the potential for lunacy was unsettling, could disturb the fragile sediments that lay just above the fevered turbulence. A mentor of mine once told me that work bound the soil of the soul.

Fatherhood was one of my vocations. *Winnie the Pooh* seemed about right for now.

-6-

In the morning, I left early to have time to visit Mom before going to my office. It was five days since the stroke story began. I was trying to maneuver past the intimate and personal on this, to some other plateau where I could function more efficiently. My tendencies trapped me in a small box, the self-blame and retribution still operational, but I knew what to do.

I saw some minuscule rays of light emanating from a variety of sources. I could cure her, for example; or pursue that goal with such ardor as to lose myself in the process. I could seek the help of others more expert in the disease that might be able to aid her. This would at least assuage me. If nothing worked and she remained an invalid, perhaps the knowledge that TPA was not a cure-all and involved risk and potential complication would ease my burden.

I walked into the ICU, and she was still asleep. I called out her name and for a moment she awoke. This was momentous to me. She opened her eyes, nodded and smiled, and then drifted back into sleep.

"Momma," I called out again, but there was no answer. And, as my spirits rose, so did they fall, but I was growing accustomed to this, something hardening within me toward the whole brutal affair, the earliest stages of a protective callous forming, as my mother had formed in her own difficult life. I called her name once more but to no avail. What was the process at work here? Why the profound slumber that did not stir? I knew the answer but still wondered when she would awaken.

Dr. Regan, the internist, walked in. "How are you, Rick," he asked.

Regan was an excellent internist, trusted by everyone. At any given time, he may have between 20 and 30 very sick patients in house he was caring for, including several in the ICU. The emergency room, anesthesia, family doctors, and surgeons consulted him regularly.

He walked around to my mother's side, pulling out his stethoscope. He listened to her heart and lungs. He then looked at the flashing lights of the monitor above her head: the numbers and squiggles, accompanied by the steady beeping that coincided with the beating of her heart.

The nurse walked in with my mother's chart. She opened the flow sheet that contained the hour-by-hour account of my mother's clinical course. She wanted to say something but stopped. She, too, looked at the monitor screen. The three of us stood there saying nothing, as if mesmerized by the green numbers and squiggles, attended by the regular cadence of the beeping, at once annoying yet reassuring.

"She is still very sleepy, generally not responsive. But her vital signs have been stable," the nurse finally spoke.

"Good, good," Regan said. "She's getting the heparin?"

"Yes."

"Keep the IV at 100cc/hour. She's still NPO." ("nothing per os" or mouth)

I heard the words but did not react to them in any way. Instead, I continued my meditation on the monitor, enthralled somehow, although, it was hardly new to me. The emotional turmoil of the last couple of days had unearthed deposits of earlier perceptions, hostile and dangerous, yet fresh and revealing, as if going through previous stages in my development for the first time, experiencing old encounters with a new mind.

It was not entirely menacing. Instead, it was a renewal of sorts, a medical-religious epiphany, carried on the wings of tragedy and flawed character. I now perceived the monitor in a more literary, even transcendent, light. It was a blending of technology and spirit, of the universal nature of man and the woefully picayune attempts of science to scrutinize finite scraps of matter (while feverishly hoping to proclaim universal truths, a goal for which it was unsuited). I saw now the beeping lights unveiling another narrative, a great myth.

They told of the ancient verities, of the eternal rhythms that bound us; they evoked the mystery of human physiology, the movement of gas through lung, the contraction of heart muscle, the turgor of arteries. They depicted the ongoing saga of my mother's essential functions, her "vital signs," as it were, and, in so doing, revealed the trajectory of evolution, the path of eons, the accumulated knowledge locked up in a single beating heart, the source of which remained hidden from science's probing hands, but known by faith. But for all that was revealed by the beeping lights, in its regularity and meter, for all that resonated from murky paths and ancient horizons gone forever, there was much that it did not tell.

They did not tell of her mind, or her ability to raise her left hand, or her spirit. This remained a darkened preserve, hidden and obscure. Only the "vegetative" functions, that amazing foundation upon which all else depended, could be discerned. Her will to live, her joys and sorrows, her five senses, mind and intellect, her creative drive, her quest for meaning remained elsewhere, concealed for now and unknowable. But all of this unavoidably rested upon the edifice of a beating heart, gas filled alveoli, and blood pressure, and so I paid homage to it and the nurse's glib enunciation that her vital signs were indeed stable.

"She's holding her own, Rick," Regan said.

"Good," I answered. But the deeper questions remained. "Why is she still so sleepy?" I asked, as if waking from my own slumber.

"It's not uncommon. She might have some edema, some mild compression; the brain stem may not function normally. It'll take time."

The words fell upon my head like so many stones.

He felt her pulse. "Yeah, she's OK for now."

"Thanks, Bruce."

And so, I sat with my mother who communed in the darkness from which no light emerged. I held her limp hand, and thought back to another time of supreme helplessness and cruel circumstance.

There was a knock on the door, and Jerry ran to get it. "Who's there," he said. Whoozeah. And a voice answered through the door.

"Mailman."

"Hey, Ma," Jerry screamed, "it's the mailman."

"Well, open the door, for cryin' out loud!" She was in the kitchen, stirring a pot of lentils. Jack and Larry looked up from the little black and white TV in the living room. Cliff was sitting on the floor, and I was drawing some pictures of animals with a pencil and paper. I heard Jerry turn the locks and open the door. "C.O.D.," said the voice.

"Huh?" Jerry said.

"C.O.D., son. Call ya mudda," he said.

"Hey, Ma, it's C.O.D."

"Well, what is it?" Mom said.

"I got t'ree boxes," the guy said.

"It's three boxes, Ma."

Mom wiped her hands on a towel and lowered the gas. She walked down the hallway to the door. I stopped drawing and followed her.

"What is it?" Mom asked again when she got to the door.

"I got t'ree boxes, M'am, C.O.D."

"Well, how much is it?"

"Fifteen bucks."

"I don't have that kind of money," Mom said.

"Den, I can't leave 'em, M'am."

"Well, what is it?"

"Ya mean whut's inside?"

"Yeah."

"I dunno."

I looked at the three cardboard boxes stacked in the hall outside the door, rope tied around each of them, the seams covered with brown tape. Our apartment was on the third floor. He had to carry each one up individually. He was sweating in his blue uniform. I saw my mother's name on one of the boxes: "Matilda Moss, 867 Crotona Park North, Bronx, New York."

"Hey, Ma, it's got your name on it."

"Hush, Rick," she said. "Who's it from?" Mom asked the mailman.

"'Issac Moss,' from Fort Lauderdale, Florida."

"Grandpa," Mom said. 'Grandpa' was what Mom said when she meant my father's dad. She called her father 'Nono.' We hardly ever saw Grandpa. Since Dad left us, we hadn't seen him at all. We just saw Nono and Nona. I remembered Grandpa, though. He gave us quarters and rides in his car.

"Why'd he send it C.O.D.?"

"Beats me, lady."

"What's the matter with him? Doesn't he know we're broke?" She looked at Jerry and me. I shrugged. Then Larry and Jack walked over.

The mailman folded his arms, looked at Mom, and blinked a couple of times. "Jeez, lady, I dunno whuttatellya."

"*What do I do?*" *Mom seemed to ask no one in particular.*

"*I dunno, lady.*"

"*Larry, Jack, what do I do? That cheapskate! C.O.D.*"

"*I got a few dollars, Ma,*" *Larry said. Larry worked at the candy store on Boston Road after school. He might have some money. And I had two dollars saved up.*

"*What do I do?*" *Mom asked again.* "*How do I know what's in them? Maybe he sent jewelry? Or new clothes for you kids to wear? Or something for the house.*"

"*Yeah, Ma, or a baseball glove,*" *Jerry said.*

"*Or sneakers,*" *I said.*

"*Or a radio,*" *Jack said.*

"*How much didja say it was, Mister?*"

"*Fifteen bucks, lady.*"

"*Can I open the boxes first?*" *she asked.*

"*No, M'am.*"

My mother's eyes darted around. "*Oh, Lord in heaven,*" *she said.* "*Your useless father, I don't have a dime to my name. I don't know what to do.*" *She wrung her hands. She looked at the ceiling and closed her eyes. She turned to the five pairs of eyes.* "*Kids,*" *she said,* "*help me. I don't know what to do.*" *She closed her eyes again and furrowed her brow, as if thinking hard. Then she opened her eyes and said with sudden conviction,* "*Kids, give me your money. Whatever you have. Grandpa wouldn't send us junk.*"

We scrambled to the little places where we each hid our money. I opened the drawer where I kept my underwear and proudly pulled out two wrinkled one dollar bills. Larry went to his room where he had some money in a shoe. Jerry had some quarters saved up in a glass jar by his bed. Mom opened up the closet door and rifled through Dad's old jackets. Then she hurried to the chair by the TV and lifted the cushion where she hid some money. Then to an ashtray on the washing machine where she had some coins. She put the money together, counted out fifteen dollars in bills and change, and nervously handed it with both hands to the befuddled man.

"*T'anks, lady,*" *he said, numbly pocketing the small pile without bothering to check it. He carried the boxes into the house. Jack went into the kitchen and got a knife.* "*Should I open 'em, Ma?*"

"*Here, let me do it.*"

Mom cut the rope of the first box, and then along the seam, splitting the tape. She pulled the leaves of the box, cut further along the inner fold, and finally spread the box open. There was crumbled newspaper packed inside, which Mom threw out. We could see some folded material and old clothes. Old pants, shirts, and socks. The shirts were white but actually yellow because they were old. The clothing had a damp, mildewed smell. There were little white balls that had a funny odor.

"*Moth balls,*" *Larry said. Mom stared at the old clothes, blinking.*

"*He must be senile,*" *she muttered under her breath nervously. She quickly went to the next box and opened it. She licked her lips anxiously and clicked her tongue. We watched, hoping the box would have something new, something wrapped and pinned, like a new shirt, or a new pair of socks or underwear, or a toy, or something. Mom pulled out more crumbled newspaper, and we each fought to get a look, ready to grab something if it looked like it might be for us. Then we smelled the same moldy odor.*

I wondered why Grandpa sent us his old clothes, which wouldn't fit anyway. Mom pulled out the yellowed shirts, the pants with lint on them, some suspenders and belts, and faded long underwear. She held each item out to see what it was and then folded it up and placed them neatly in a pile on the floor. None of us said anything, and Mom went over to the third box. She cut uneasily with the sharp knife, and I worried she might hurt herself. She opened it and found some magazines, old books, a few pencils and erasers, pajamas, underwear, and a pair of wrinkled beat-up shoes. She held them up, looking at them. She stacked the magazines on the floor and put the old shoes on top. She looked around at the piles of clothing, the three boxes ripped open, the magazines, books, and the cruddy, smelly shoes.

Mom tried to control herself but could not. She held her hands to her face and began sobbing. We stood there at first, all five kids watching her. Then, one by one, each of us began crying, as if it were contagious, filling the whole house with weeping. Mom ignored us, still crying into her hands. And the chorus of lamentations continued.

Then, Mom stopped crying. She stood up and looked at the clothing. She began holding them up against her kids to see if anything fit. None of it did, nor did any of it look good. Then she came to the shoes. She sized them up before deciding that something had to come from all this. She handed them to Jack. She didn't check to see if they fit or if he liked them. She said, "These are yours." And Jack had to wear Grandpa's old shoes because Mom spent fifteen hard-earned bucks to get some worthless, moldy clothing, and something had to be salvaged.

Then Mom told us to clean everything up and throw the crappy clothes and boxes in the garbage. She went back to the kitchen to finish her lentils.

I left my mother in the ICU and went over to my office. I called the hospital librarian to get the NINDS article and other more recent pieces on stroke. There would be more current studies since NINDS, and it would be useful to see how the original findings on TPA stood up over time. It is common that a single landmark article will make a big splash, not just in the medical community, but in the general media where the daily grind of the 24-hour news cycle demanded regular material to sensationalize (with or without merit) – and TPA and other clot busters had made quite a stir.

I remembered reading something about it in *Time* or *Newsweek*. It had first been featured because of its notoriety with acute myocardial infarctions (heart attacks), for which clinicians found useful. Then came the NINDS study, the seminal article that established TPA as a viable treatment for reversing strokes. As with many important studies, there may have been an initial overreaction to the primary trial; further such studies may not show the same results; complications may appear or less salutary outcomes, forcing a reassessment of the original results, if not an outright rejection of them. This was the self-correcting nature of scientific inquiry, an essential feature.

I completed my day in the office, still a struggle. I remained morose but not fully lost. If I could probe this matter intelligently, I could, perhaps, undo the hopeless blunder and move forward from the self-loathing that had possessed me since the event. I sat for a moment at my desk, covered in the same morass of mail that invaded my office everyday. What a hysterical nation this was, the obscene amounts of ink, paper, and postage wasted to convince other Americans that they desperately needed another credit card or long distance service. I ran through the pile, discarding two thirds of it.

I heard the phone ring and saw my private line light up. It would be for me. I let the women in the front answer it anyway. Maureen, my office manager, called on the intercom and told me it was my brother Cliff, the youngest of the five boys. I had left a message for him a day or so ago. It was not avoidance that kept me from informing him or my other brothers sooner; only I wanted to see how Mom was progressing, especially after the first day when it seemed only minor. I picked up the private line.

"Hey, yo, Breeze," I said, shifting instantly into our usual New York guttural mode. My New York accent was never thick and, after ten years in Indiana, had all but disappeared. Not so, Cliff. His nickname from the Bronx was Cool Breeze, a label that definitely suited him and certainly his own self-image. He had become the tough guy of the family, smoked, had a big tattoo on his right upper arm, and managed a garment factory in Manhattan. He had a high school equivalency diploma, which meant nothing to him. The world was still his oyster, and he dripped with macho confidence, although not in an annoying way. He lived in Brooklyn with his Italian wife and two kids.

"Hey, Ricky, so what's going on?"

"Ya heard about Ma?"

"Yeah, Ying told me she had a stroke. I just talked to her. When'd it happen?"

"Four days ago."

"I can't believe it." I heard the anger rising in his voice. "An' you're only tellin' me about it now?"

"I-"

"Whatchya do ta her?"

"I-I didn't do . . . "

"She's at your house for a frickin' week, an' she's got a stroke."

"You don't get a stroke from a one week visit!" I said.

"You're so damn smart, we know all about it. Mom's been tellin' us for years. I jus' know she goes to your house for a week, an' she comes out wit' a stinkin' stroke!"

"You want to listen for a minute, and I'll tell you what happened," I said.

"'An' whyda take so frickin' long callin' me?"

"Would you take it easy! I'm here taking care of Mom, and you're-"

"Takin' care of Mom, *sure* you are . . ."

"You got a big mouth, Cliff!"

"Ah, kiss off, Rick. So stinkin' smart all dese years."

I gave him the last obnoxious word. He loved his mother; I knew that. He was the youngest and had his own special relationship with her. He called her regularly, had her over his place in Brooklyn often, always paying for the taxi both ways. He was generous to everyone, especially her. He could scarcely imagine my own inner melt down. I was glad I had not called him before.

"Alright. So whutdahell happened?" he said finally.

"She had a stroke. And she's not doing well. Four days ago. At my place. We got her over to the hospital, started her on some blood thinner. At first, it didn't look bad. The next morning she was moving her extremities. I figured it was a minor stroke, and she'd be out of the hospital in a few days."

"Then?"

"Then it progressed."

"Howdahell did dat happen?"

"The stroke wound up involving a bigger part of the brain."

"Can't dey keep dat from happenin'?" He was getting close now to the dirty little secret. The whole conversation was like an open wound.

"Yeah, but it doesn't always work," I said, avoiding the issue.

"So what's goin' on now?"

"She's in the Intensive Care Unit."

"Ahh, Jeez."

"Her vital signs are stable, her heart's OK. But she had a dense stroke, she can't move her left side."

"She's paralyzed?"

"Yeah, the left side is out. She can't get up or move around. Can't eat. She's got a feeding tube. It's not good."

"Can't get outta bed?"

"No, she's bedridden," I said.

"Oh crap, she must be goin' nuts."

"She sleeps most of the time."

"But is she able to speak?"

"Not much right now, but that should get better. It was a right-sided stroke, so it didn't affect the speech centers."

"But will she be able to get up and move around?"

"It's too early to tell."

"Crap, an' she was so strong, like a horse, could walk for miles." I listened to my brother go through the same process I had, the disbelief and the anger. "She was in good health, right? She had nuttin' wrong wit' her."

"Usual things. Some cholesterol, some diabetes, and she's 78," I said.

"Yeah, but she was sooo healthy before – strong as an ox."

"I know."

"Really sucks. I'm so glad I had her over my house da day before she left, had a good time wit' da kids, spent da whole damn day tagedda. She was healt'y as a horse, could walk for miles."

"I know, it's a shock. I'll never forget the day it happened, last Saturday, we were going to have Labor Day weekend together. I was looking forward to it. It's so beautiful now, too, weather's perfect."

"And 'dis crap can happen jus' like dat?"

"Yeah."

"No warnin', nuttin'."

"Yeah, just like that."

"I taut she was good fa anudda ten years."

"So did I."

"Crap! Nona lasted 'till she was 96. It's like we're gettin' gypped."

"I know."

"Really sucks. How's she takin' it? She depressed?"

"I can't really tell, she just comes in and out of it for a few seconds and then she's sleeping again."

"'Dat's normal?"

"Yeah, for now," I said.

"Like a frickin' invalid."

"Yeah. So let the brothers know. And the aunts and uncles."

"I still can't believe dis crap."

The phone call bothered me. His reaction though was understandable. The bad humors, though, returned once more. My patients needed my attention, but I could not concentrate, each encounter tedious and difficult. I observed myself weakening. It was all a matter of steps, an irresistible force somehow seductive, yet suicidal. This was madness, I realized, crystallized and defined. Such was the effect of my impasse. It was a cruel punishment to be inept when one generally enjoyed glowing self-impressions. I had recrudesced -

the disease process upon me again, another spasm of self-blame.

But enough! How feeble I was! I could not see past the dereliction of a lifetime, my failure to act, the fate of my mother hanging around my neck. How to justify my lapse and restore meaning to my pathetic life? How to navigate safely, with some reasonable balance of emotions? By *will*? For this was all I had to hold the ailing enterprise together. Wretched thoughts! Be gone! I must reconcile my imbecility. How? Work, yes, and research. And what else? I did not know. How dependent were our two fates, I thought. My mother and I. I could not bear to contemplate her demise at my untrustworthy hands. I felt my tenuous self slipping into despair.

I went to the ICU. My mother still slept deeply. She opened her eyes briefly and then closed them, preferring to commune with the angels than with her miserable son. I sat and observed her. The monitor over her bed exchanged only pleasantries today, reassuring squiggles and beeps that attested to her fine fettle. For some twisted reason, I decided to feel her pulse. I placed my first two fingers over the soft part of her wrist, just to the side of her tendon. I then sought out the workman-like pulse of her radial artery. It was coy at first, but then revealed itself. It throbbed and relaxed rhythmically, corresponding to the beating of her heart, not a timid or hesitant beat at all, but giddy and confident. It also beat in synchrony with the beeping of the monitor, a perfect mingling of the sciences, physiology and medical technology, the latter dutifully tracking the former in wondrous tandem. I sat by her side, fingers on her warm wrist, immersed in her essential rhythm, imagining her pulse, the pulse that bespoke of her heart, the heart that had never failed her. It had not always been tears and misery. I remember . . .

In summers, we went to Orchard Beach, near City Island, in the Bronx. We took the number 20 bus to Fordham road and then the 12 bus to Orchard Beach. I was with Cliff and Jerry, holding the blankets. Larry and Jack, the two older ones, did not come. Jerry had the thermos with orange juice and my mother had the bag with the peanut butter and jelly sandwiches. She sat opposite us, watching us, a soft smile on her face. She seemed happy, finding pleasure in her three young children.

The bus was crowded. I could smell the sun tan oil on everyone. The other passengers wore sandals, shorts, and t-shirts, carrying blankets, thermoses, and beach chairs, some listened to their transistor radios, holding onto handrails or sitting quietly. We exited the bus and walked over to the beach, the bright sun, the smell of the ocean, and the warm breeze upon us. The boardwalk was actually not of wood, like the one at Rockaway Beach in Queens, but of large tiles that became hot as the day progressed. There was a concession stand, first aid center, police station, and a loudspeaker that made announcements about kids being lost or a car parked in the wrong place. We walked to Section 11 (my mother's favorite) and onto the sand, which was even hotter than the boardwalk.

"I told you kids to keep your sneakers on," Mom said. We found a spot, not too crowded. We checked the sand before spreading the blanket to make sure there was no horse crap (from horses police rode on patrol).

"It's OK, Ma," Jerry said, "there's no horsecrap."

"Watch your mouth," Mom said.

We put sneakers on each corner of the blanket so the wind wouldn't blow it, and then the food, thermos, and towels. We took off our shorts with our bathing suits on underneath, so we didn't have to go to the lockers or have Mom hold a towel around us while we changed on the beach. Jerry and I ran to the water, excited by the sea, the blue sky, the piercing white sand. We dove headlong into it and splashed and frisked for the next hour.

Mom walked leisurely in her bathing suit, holding Cliff's hand; he was still too young to go by himself. She sat in the shallow water with Cliff nearby, letting the gentle waves wash over her, playing with Cliff who desperately wanted to frolic with his older brothers but could not. Mom relaxed as she watched over us, enjoying the warm breeze and the sun on her face.

Later, Mom called us for lunch. We resisted at first, but relented, feeling hungry. We walked to our blanket. "Dry yourselves, kids," Mom said. We sat down while Mom opened the thermos and unwrapped the peanut butter and jelly sandwiches. She cut up some peaches and gave each of us a slice. We sat contentedly as Mom passed us our sandwiches and small cups of orange juice.

While eating, I noticed an Hispanic family sitting on a blanket next to ours. There was a little girl about my age, which was five, wearing a bathrobe. What interested me was that she did not have a bathing suit underneath, and she sat with her legs up. I began looking between her legs, curious what was there. We, of course, had no sisters, and so I did not know what to expect. The little girl gazed back at me quizzically. At first, I could not see anything but then she shifted her legs and I could see directly between them. I blinked at first, disbelieving. To my five-year-old mind, something seemed terribly wrong. It was just skin and a velvety crease, nothing else, a fine vertical line and delicate mounds on either side of it. The absence of any further substance or structure was almost disabling. I was convinced something horrible had happened!

They were playing Spanish music on the radio. She picked up a piece of watermelon and started eating it, spitting out the seeds. She did not look sick! Her father, mother, and brother were lying on beach towels next to her, oiled down and getting a tan. They seemed utterly at ease. I finished my sandwich and looked again. The same hairless skin and crease, like a wound. But, there was no blood. Nor did she appear to be in pain. I wiped the peach from my face with a napkin. I said to Jerry, "There's something the matter with that girl!"

"Huh?" Jerry said.

"That girl, there's something the matter with her."

"How do you know?"

"I can tell."

"Whaddaya mean? Tell what?"

I walked over to her.

"Are you OK," I asked. She had black eyes and long dark brown hair. She had watermelon juice all over her face. "What's the matter with you?" I inquired again.

She wiped her face with the sleeve of her white bathrobe and stared at me.

"How come you don't have anything there?"

She didn't answer. Her mother, who was on her stomach, lifted herself onto her elbows. She had big breasts like Mom. "Que pasa?" she said.

"What's the matter with your daughter, she doesn't have anything?"

"Que?"

"She doesn't have anything down there?"

The mother nudged the father. He was chubby and hairy. He was holding a folded aluminum panel under his face for tanning. "Aiyyy, que pasa," I heard him say as he rolled over. He sat up reluctantly, his belly hanging over his bathing suit. "Hola, niño."

"There's somethin' the matter with your daughter."

"She looks OK to me, amigo," he said.

"Yeah, but she doesn't have anything down there."

"Down where?"

"Between her legs."

He narrowed his eyes.

"There's just some skin an' a line there, she doesn't have a penis."

His wife sat up.

They both glared at me. But then the father sort of sniffed and shook his head. "Ees that your mother, niño?"

"Uh huh."

By now, Mom was walking over. "This girl doesn't have a penis, Ma."

"What?" Mom said, almost choking. "Ricky what are you saying?" She looked at me with shock, as if I had committed a grievous sin. By now, though, the father was chuckling, and soon my mother began to smile. Then she started laughing. "Ricky, you crazy kid, what's the matter with you." And then to the family, "I'm so sorry," but by now there didn't seem to be anything to apologize for. The only ones who weren't laughing were the girl and me. I still didn't know what was so funny since the girl obviously had something wrong with her.

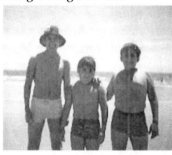

"Eet ees no problem, miss," the father said, and Mom put a comforting hand over my shoulder and guided me back to our blanket.

When Jerry heard the story, he called me an idiot. "Shuddup," I said.

-8-

When I got home from the office that evening, my kids greeted me. They heard the door open, a familiar sound, then the closet door open as I hung my jacket. Then, I heard the stampede of little feet running toward me, followed by, "Daddyyyyyyy." And with this, Arielle and Noah came hurtling into me as if I were an inanimate object, bursting into my arms as small projectiles, fully expecting, as was the tradition, to be lifted and kissed. This was a balm for me, my conventional routines rescuing me. How odd, it seemed, that I, the former radical, should become so inured to the habits of middle class life. I picked up my two hamsters, Noah, in his shorts, and Arielle, in her pretty tank top.

"Daddy did you bring us something," Arielle asked, her brown locks rolling down upon her face and shoulders, her cheeks bunched up like small nuggets, as lovely a face as I should ever hope to see.

"Well, yes, how did you know?" I said in a mocking tone, since I brought something home everyday. She shrugged innocently and giggled, and I was smitten once more, shaken from my reveries by this delicate, smiling creature who knew nothing of my worries, only knew of her Daddy who came home each evening, bearing small gifts and favors, the highlight of her day, and mine as well.

Noah, not to be outdone, forced himself into our little circle. "What about me, Daddy," he said, a pout forming on his face, the soft skin furrowing, his lips pursing. It was an attractive face, a pleasing mix of the orient and occident, his eyes with just a trace of angularity, enough to make him intriguing; he combed his chestnut hair straight back, my little Adonis.

"Oh, of course, did you think Daddy would forget his little boy?" The pout vanished and a golden smile appeared, a piercing light, and little white glistening ivories materialized just beyond his tapered lips. Everyone was content now because Daddy was back and brandishing treats. I kissed each of them and placed them on the floor and then reached into my left pocket within which lay two gumballs I bought each day on the way out of the medical office building. I took them out, cupped my two hands around them, and shook them, making a rattling sound that brought smiles.

"Oh, me, Daddy, let me pick," Arielle said. They battled, as was typical, over first choice. Although the two items were identical they fought anyway, their unfortunate rivalry extending into the most absurd arenas.

"No, me, Daddy," said Noah, the two now jockeying intensely. Here, I could only lose, because someone would pick first and the other would sulk. Noah, as he was prone to, resolved the dilemma by slipping his hand in before any further discussion and absconding with one of the pieces, dashing off before I could stop him.

Arielle protested but only mildly. "Noah!" she said, a refrain I heard often, his antics already legendary, but being older she whined less and was content with her piece of gum anyway, so the foul mood dissipated quickly.

With the major decisions of the moment thusly decided, I stepped out of my shoes and into my slippers and walked into the house, holding Arielle's hand. I actually seemed to be smiling; such was the power of these two upon me.

Ying was next in line, and, indeed, she was dressed in tight blue shorts and white blouse, cut low, revealing sizeable cleavage for this small Asian woman. She looked up from the stove, a CD of Itzhak Perlman playing traditional Jewish music from Eastern Europe in the background. She had become quite a Jew since converting several years ago. It was something for a Thai Buddhist to flip into the Jewish fold, the two cultures and religions as alien as could be. I insisted and so she studied the prayer books, learned our customs, immersed herself in the *mikvah* (the ritual bath), appeared before the congregation, and announced that she was honored to become "one of the children of Israel."

The congregation was delighted for this was something novel, Christian conversions being the routine, and Asian Buddhist cameos, as it were, something of an anomaly. They also loved her "acceptance" speech. I had helped write it, but she had read it well and with much ardor. She then recited the *Shema* (Judaism's most sacred prayer) while standing behind the *bimah* (the Torah lectern in the synagogue). So now, in my home, we listened to Itzhak Perlman playing traditional Jewish music. In my naïveté, I had hoped her conversion would bring her closer to my mother. Unfortunately, it did not.

Ying was busy stirring up a dish of tofu and broccoli with peanut sauce, a Thai favorite. She placed a kiss upon my lips and said, "Hi, Dad," as was her custom, and this, too, was helpful, a kind of mild stimulant. It seemed, unwittingly, as if a conspiracy was afoot within my home to awaken me from my deep slumbers. Whether it was deliberate or not or just my acute awareness of every abrasive detail around me, I did not know. But, it was effective and seemed to stir me from this craggy pothole into which I had fallen – a fallow place indeed.

"Hello, sweetheart, how are you?" I said, enjoying the familiar tapestry of soothing home life, yet with the recollection of my mother pressing in on the margins.

"Are you ready to eat," Ying asked.

"Yeah, let me go up and change my clothes."

When I returned there was a spinach and tomato salad with Italian vinaigrette, rice, and the tofu and broccoli in peanut sauce, which smelled wonderful, better than a restaurant. It was oral gratification, nothing more, a step backwards through the stages of life, returning to the earliest and most primitive, to soothe my wounds. I sat down, and Arielle brought me a magazine. I smiled and gave her a little kiss, and then she went to play with her brother. Ying sat down next to me. I placed a spoonful of food in my mouth.

"How's your mother?" she asked.

"About the same."

"Is she waking up at all?"

"Very little. Still sleeping mostly, but stable," I said.

"What did the doctor say?"

"Takes time, not much else. She barely responds when I walk in, so I just sit with her."

"Does he think she can recover?" she asked.

"He can't say. We have to wait."

"Is there anything else we can do?"

"Just our prayers."

"Are there any new treatments?" she asked.

"I'm sure there are therapies and rehab and all sorts of things we'll be getting into, but she's just not ready for it yet."

I sipped some wine. "Did Jerry call?" I asked.

"About an hour ago."

I had some salad. "Was he angry?"

"No, but Cliff was when he called," she said.

"I know. I spoke to him. He blamed me for causing the stroke."

"Your brothers may resent you, Rick."

"What'd Cliff say to you when he called?" I asked.

"He asked me what I did to his mother."

"What did you say?"

"I told him I didn't do anything to his mother." I was very angry.

"How was Jerry?" I asked.

"He was fine."

"So, he wasn't angry about my not calling him right away?"

"No, I think he understood. I tried to explain to him how you felt." Ying and Jerry were good friends. He was Ying's ally in the family. When she had an argument with me, she called Jerry. That's because Jerry always managed to see me in the worst possible light. Ying's complaints seemed to serve his purposes, although it hadn't always been that way. I used to protect Jerry, defended him when he was on drugs and when he lived in the "Ashram," a yoga commune in upstate New York where he lived five years. Since the Ashram days, he had become quite a success in the insurance field, a big name in a big company, an amazing turnaround and something, by the way, I was intensely proud of. But with that unexpected success came a surprising competitiveness that I had never observed before.

I continued with the tofu and broccoli. Despite everything, I was feeling better. Ying moved her chair closer to me and rubbed my neck. "Call Jerry later," she said. "They want to visit."

I kept eating as she massaged my shoulders. I had always loved eating. I continued in this quest for peace through eating, as if I had not ingested for days. Something had broken within me, a sudden burst of neuronal activity creating a bath of favorable chemi-

cal mediators, the effect of which was to produce some
semblance of inner tranquility. How I arrived at this,
I had no idea, but I relished it just the same. I felt en-
ergized, and, yet, paradoxically, calm. Had my wife
spiked the food?

I suddenly longed for my study. I wanted to read
more about stroke, its mechanism, its unseemly habits, and the tripwire finnickiness of the brain. I excused
myself.

"It was delicious, sweetheart, thanks." She looked
at me sideways. She was growing accustomed to my
weird behavior of late. "I'll call Jerry later." I went into
my study. The kids were playing outside. I had time.

I sat down in the leather chair and strummed
through the pages. I came upon the dog-eared page I
had marked. There were pen marks, underlined passages, and little asterisks in the margins. It was all so
dry and dusty. It was science, after all, not poetry. For
me though, it had taken on more the dimension of a
detective story. It fascinated me, despite my biases. I
analyzed the tiny cellular and molecular villains that
filled the broad canvas of the disease, a corrupted vision that compelled me even as I despised it.

I wanted to find out more about the *platelet,* this ridiculous fragment that seemed very much at the center
of things, at the center of the process of stroke. There
would be much to say about this little particle, I was
sure, for even from the cloistered domains in which I
wandered, as an otolaryngologist, I, and everyone in
medicine, knew of this tiny beast from which so much
good and so much bad arose; of the vast array of cu-
ratives and antidotes that had been created to rein in
its madness and diminish its effect. I gazed almost in
amusement at the pages, the dark etchings against a
vacuous white background, holding an intolerable degree of technical detail concerning molecules and enzymes and factors. I stared out my window for a mo-

ment. Green and summery, the season still in evidence, the filtered golden light fashioning elongated shadows as the sun began its final descent. I felt weary in pursuit of painful subjects long forgotten (not reviewed since the distant days of medical school), the domain of others who had to understand the complex sequences so they may minister properly.

I had gone in other directions in my career. I could not tolerate the dense jungles of the neurologic sciences, yet I found myself now eagerly clambering up and down its trunks and branches, savoring its fragrances and resins and happily so, even insanely so, as if obsessed. I at once hated and lusted for it, a freakish disorder, filled with greed and remorse, overtaken by some heinous urge to possess and dominate it, as unholy and blasphemous as it was, as obtuse as any medical treatise could be. The exalted facade of science again beckoned, such a constricted apparatus, so sickening and weary – but essential. I began. The sequence of events was as follows:

Somewhere in a branch of the right middle cerebral artery of my mother's brain, a microscopic rupture of a plaque occurred within the lumen (the "inside") of the vessel itself. The ruptured plaque, with its underbelly exposed to the blood rushing by, teeming with essential life components (red blood cells, lymphocytes, enzymes, and the like), began to attract a collection of platelets. Then more and more gathered, until there were thousands, millions, gathering, all following their ancient mandates, bound by the cryptic code contained within their DNA, guided by a complex algorithm of chemical affinities, swarming ravenously like locusts.

I allowed myself to slip into a poetic reverie of the otherwise appalling scientific description - for the problem was infinitely more arcane than the crumb metaphor I had used for my daughter.

The platelet was a rather inconsequential little jot, less than a single cell, a mere fragment, a piece of cellular debris, a miniscule bag of cytoplasm, devoid even of a nucleus, disfigured and incomplete from birth. It was the daughter of an even more bizarre freak known as the *megakaryocyte,* a bloated polyploid monster that lacked a defined nucleus, possessing instead full complements of DNA floating around in its cytoplasm, hence its psychotic "multipolarity." This megakaryocyte gave birth to platelets by a kind of "calving" process. It sloughed a piece of itself off with the requisite membrane systems, organelles, and granules needed for the orphaned platelet to carry on. The platelet, in turn, meandered mindlessly through the bloodstream guided by its own sliver of DNA, focused solely on its penchant for damaged vessels.

And yet, within this pathetic fragment lay a sophisticated biochemical apparatus capable of manufacturing an astonishing assortment of proteins, receptors, and enzymes all committed to the single task of recognizing damaged vessels and sealing them, a critical player in the clotting system. With such an inventory, the platelet could detect collagen from a damaged vessel, alter its shape, adjust and enhance its receptors, activate other platelets, and release an array of coagulation molecules, including fibrinogen and thrombin, which resulted in the formation of a clot. The initial small collection of platelets became an aggregate, which became a thrombus, which became an occlusion (a blockage): the lumen of the vessel choked by platelets stuffed in a meshwork of fibrin, thereby shutting off circulation. A stroke.

The ramifications of this wizardry were apparent. I nearly shuddered as I contemplated the process unfolding within my mother. I continued.

The clotting system balanced precariously on the precipice between activation and inhibition, an amazingly finely tuned equilibrium that kept the peace, maintaining the normal fluidity of the blood stream, but utterly primed and ready to catapult into thrombus formation with the slightest provocation, at exactly the right time and in precisely the right place. Clotting involved a multitude of cells, proteins, receptors, cofactors, and the like, all poised to play their role in a dizzying choreography. And our tiny proletarian, the platelet, with its undistinguished pedigree, played the lead role. It was both hero and antihero, absolutely essential to life as we knew it, preventing catastrophic hemorrhage in case of injury, yet tragically implicated in the process of thrombogenic (vascular) disease, causing heart attacks and strokes: a stupid cell, if you will, incapable of distinguishing between a vessel torn by trauma and one ruptured by an atherosclerotic plaque. As such, it had become the central character in the greatest disease process of our times: vascular disease, which killed and maimed by the millions yearly – a holocaust.

I pushed back from the desk and again sought comfort in my window. It was getting dark, the temperature cooling with the arrival of night. I saw the lights of the house across the street turn on. Then the street lamps. Then darkness, the sky dressed in velvety, black cords. The kids were outside playing. I could hear them, their voices like small clarinets. They roused me, their squeals and laughter, their delight at nothing. I stood and looked out. The cool air felt good. September was perfect, but the universe configured against me. The calm sky was wretched, like a nagging wound. Let me find solace in my children.

I put my little friends (the kids) to sleep, and I sat down with Ying in the living room on the sofa opposite the piano. Across from me were standing lamps and an ornate console with a picture of my mother on it. It was my favorite photo of her, and I had it enlarged and framed. She was hoisting a glass of wine and had a great smile, taken, no doubt, at one of our many family occasions years ago, perhaps a bar mitzvah or wedding. It captured perfectly her passion and joy. I said nothing to Ying who seemed content with the local newspaper.

I went to bed, praying for a decent sleep. I did not get it, the meddlesome little alarm announcing itself far too soon. As I awakened, I did so with the overwhelming wish that I could simply disappear. It all seemed so tenuous, the shenanigans of survival, the pageantry (outward display that were of necessity dishonest) and spectacle of carving out an existence. It had been years since I had felt this way. The exigencies of life had kept me far from it. I was the son of my mother who taught me to endure.

The last time I wanted to disappear, I had read about the *Idealists* and their notion that reality existed only within the mind, that we were, all of us, prisoners of our sense organs and could not truly know anything. Our perceptions, they argued, did not reflect reality, only the inner workings of the mind. Everything, in other words, was an ongoing dream and true reality was unknowable.

How to prove or disprove such a thing? It was all rather frightening and threw my whole psyche into disarray. The world suddenly became unreal, more phantom than prosaic.

If reality was perception, an arrangement of neural impulses transmitted to the brain and decoded into some impression or image, then how could I know anything? It rather struck at the very core of things, did it not? I had moved deeply into the realm of the mind, a fractured, disjointed domain, and almost went insane trying to reassemble it. I sought desperately to prove that existence endured without my awareness, that events transpired quite separate and distinct from me, although the centrality and God-like features one assumed with the other solipsistic, self-centered view held a certain appeal if one got used to it.

But no, I decided to return to the parochial notion that what I perceived with my senses did indeed exist and that I could respond to these ghosts and apparitions in good conscience. If I added to this discussion, the bruising awareness I now held of stroke and its implications, the argument that perception was reality all but evaporated. Perception, thought, memory, and consciousness were all firmly rooted in the hardware of our central nervous system as evidenced by the tragic reality of stroke. (Amidst the vast sea of chemicals and nerve fibers, I also wondered, was there room for the soul?)

I pushed through the morning rituals, brushing my teeth, shaving, showering, the regularity and mindlessness of the routines, somehow helpful, a kind of glue that managed to bond the scattered elements of my being together. I did my morning yoga and push-ups, put on my clothing, combed my hair, applied cologne, and a touch of olive oil, an old secret to maintain youthful skin. By this time, Ying was stirring. The kids, who had snuck into our room at night, huddled under the blankets, sleeping soundly. She asked me how I felt. "Terrible," I said. Perhaps, I did not show it, because she told me I did not look too bad. I walked downstairs to the kitchen. Ying put on her bathrobe and followed me down. She cut me a slice of apple. I kissed her goodbye and went to work.

When I entered my office, the staff members were already busy, sitting before their computer terminals, punching keyboards, calling insurance companies, answering the phones, setting appointments, and preparing charts. They barely lifted their heads when I walked in, so intent were they in their efforts. My office manager, Beth, a middle-aged woman, looked up momentarily to mutter a brief good morning.

It was always maddening at the beginning of the day, hectic with patients, the phone, the many charts to review. There were biopsy reports, medicines, and lab results to call in. Dosages to adjust. Patients or family members with questions or problems. Applications for leave of absence or disability forms to fill out. Operative reports to send to insurance companies. Precertifications for scheduled procedures. Dictated letters to read and sign. The paperwork involved in running a medical office was overwhelming, and I was in no mood for it. I walked past my nurse, Janet. She was preparing the exam rooms and smiled just briefly before hurrying by.

I walked into my personal office. The clutter on my desk was appalling. The pile of junk mail, journals, magazines, and glossy notices was typical, which made it no less offensive. I moved past my statue of a standing Tara, a bronze Tibetan statue on a pedestal. I glanced at the woodcarvings on my walls from Burma and the mask from Guatemala. A Buddha statue adorned my desk, which itself was a beautiful dark cherry wood. There was a large plant by the window in need of watering. Two cushioned chairs and then an elegantly embroidered couch lay opposite the desk. I sat down in my leather swivel chair, the kind of chair I never imagined myself owning, and confronted the unhappy stack.

Something caught my eye: a copy of an article from a medical journal. Just then Janet, my nurse, walked in. She smiled. Such a lovely woman, she had soft, luminous, white hair and she had been to the beauty parlor. Her face was warm and friendly. She had on red lipstick, wore pearl earrings, and a white nurse's uniform. She had become a nurse at age 62 after 30 years of teaching, and the qualities she brought to her job were invaluable. Approaching seventy, she remained vibrant and indispensable.

"The article you wanted came in today on the fax."

"Yeah, I see it, thanks."

I picked it up, quickly read the abstract, and then thumbed through the pages. This was the article that launched a thousand ships. Whether we should have given the TPA was no longer a relevant consideration. The period for making that decision was three hours after the stroke. We were now six days past that, and so the discussion was purely academic. But, I was tangled in my emotions and consumed by guilt. I had a half hour before my first patient and read it in its entirety. When I finished, I felt worse. I wanted to call someone. Jason, some neurology big shot at the Med Center, the Mayo Clinic, anyone. The red light on my phone was flashing. Then a voice on the intercom. "Dr. Moss, your brother, Jerry, is calling."

-9-

At lunch, I walked over to the hospital to see Mom, aggravated by Jerry's call. Already he was pushing, as if recovering from a stroke was like selling an insurance policy. But stroke was not like closing a sale. It was more a game of attrition and agonizing delay, and Jerry did not operate that way. Everything was a frontal assault with him. And quick. Had to be quick. God bless him, he had come far with that attitude, but it would not work here. I knew that he and all the brothers were worried.

When I got to the ICU, the nurses were sitting down eating lunch. One was checking a monitor, preparing to make a call. Another looked up to tell me she had moved Mom to telemetry. I supposed this represented progress. Telemetry was a step down from the ICU in the crisis hierarchy, a unit where she could be closely monitored, although not as closely as the ICU. The nurse-to-patient ratio was lower, less than the one-to-one ratio in the ICU. Cardiac patients were frequent guests in telemetry, or anyone who needed closer monitoring than the regular floor could provide. As I walked out, the nurse mentioned that Mom was having an "echocardiogram" or ultrasound of the heart.

I entered her room just down the hall and saw a large piece of equipment next to her bed. It had dials and switches on it and a small screen, like something you might see in a submarine, which was, after all,

74

where ultrasound originated. The screen, of course, was an oscilloscope, which imaged the "echoes." There were other pieces of equipment, including a generator, a recorder, and a long probe held by the technician who was getting ready to begin the procedure. She nodded when I walked in, a little uncomfortable perhaps, with me suddenly in the room. Mom remained oblivious, still in a deep sleep.

"Who ordered this?" I asked.

"Dr. Regan," she said.

"What for?"

"To check her heart. Probably looking for a thrombus."

"Thrombus?"

"A blood clot."

"I know what a thrombus is," I said, annoyed for no reason. "You mean something in the heart that is throwing off emboli?"

"Yes," she said a little defensively.

"What's the usual source?"

"The left atrium."

I looked at the EKG monitor above the bed. Normal sinus rhythm. "She's not in atrial fibrillation."

"No, Dr. Regan was just checking."

It was one of the countless studies that internists tended to order: "fleas," I remember them being called in medical school. They checked everything, a veritable feast of studies, labs, and X-rays that issued from their sweeping pens. An ultrasound would not hurt anyway, a non-invasive study, and, who knows, maybe he would find something. The improbable object of his affection was a thrombus or thrombogenic source within the heart. And from this source, a suspect – a lowly crumb that may have broken off and *embolized*, or swam amidst the fishes of the blood stream to lodge somewhere in my mother's brain.

The technician placed some gel on my mother's chest and guided the probe over her sternum. She was firing off sound waves ("ultrasound") that passed through the chest, hit the various structures of the heart and bounced back, creating a signal or "echo" on the oscilloscope. I watched my mother slumbering, her silver hair brushed back, exposing her broad forehead with the familiar scar on the right side that she suffered in a car accident. They had sewn it up unevenly, creating a slight ridge.

The nurse looked at the oscilloscope and made some adjustments, turning a dial here and there. She placed the probe on the left side of my mother's chest, slicing the heart, if you will, horizontally, with yet another beam of silent sound. She looked at the oscilloscope and mumbled something about this being the "parasternal long axis view." Whatever it was, she liked it and hit a switch to record the findings.

Mom remained somnolent as ultrasonic waves bombarded her chest. The nurse slid the probe to another point on her sternum and fired off more volleys. I watched the process, curious but detached. The room was dimly lit and windowless. How depressing. I wanted to rouse my mother and walk out. I did not like the darkness or her unending sleep. And now, this miserable echocardiogram. She had no cardiac history. What was the purpose? The nurse continued plumbing the depths of Mom's chest, recording the echoes, searching the chambers of her heart for a thrombus, some explanation for the terrible accident that had occurred.

I began to wonder. If a thrombus had formed in Mom's heart, battered as it would have been by her left atrium, what sort of journey would a fragment broken off from that thrombus have had to undertake to have caused her stroke? This otherwise harmless speck would have fractured off and traversed the mitral valve, leaving the left atrium and entering the left ventricle. Here, an amazing vortex would have swept it up, a powerful sway and pitch, as the thick muscles of the heart contracted and expelled the crumb along with its fraction of blood through the aortic valve and into the aorta. From here, the speck may have traveled in any number of directions, each causing its own special disaster. But in Mom's case, to cause *her* disaster, it would have journeyed up through the right brachiocephalic artery, into the carotid artery, up through the neck, and into the cranium. Having now broached the inner sanctum, the holy of holies (the brain), it would have continued on its eventful route.

I began taking notes compulsively, outlining the blood supply of the brain, which, coincidentally, I had reviewed yesterday. I envisioned the meager crumb on its path, a tedious exercise yet one I embraced, finding solace in the detail and grand scheme. I saw crimson rivers and estuaries of blood, filtering down to ever smaller tributaries and finally to a fine filigree meshwork insinuating itself within the fevered swirls and twists of the neural elements of the brain. I saw the scarlet crests colliding against the inner walls of the vessels, the garnet plumes surging forward in triumphant waves, seeking access and orbits, penetrating deeper into the willowy labyrinth of the brain, carrying unknown its forbidden freight, the benighted crumb.

I diagrammed the crumb passing through the carotid artery, glancing off the base of the cochlea before advancing along the floor of the middle cranial fossa, sheathed in the finest dural layers and enveloped by a silken venous sack known as the cavernous sinus. The carotid coursed gracefully upward and then back into the "Circle of Willis," a vascular confluence at the base of the brain, from whence came the middle cerebral artery, the largest branch of the carotid artery and a direct continuation of it. It passed upward through the

Sylvian Fissure, the groove separating the frontal and temporal lobes of the brain, a weeping, dank chasm enclosed by the densest of circuitry, before dividing into roughly twelve branches that fanned out to supply the lateral surface of the brain.

I remembered that the middle cerebral artery also sent off perforating branches, small spear-like conduits, to supply the inner structures of the brain, and carefully penciled them in. These vessels nourished the *internal capsule,* the nerve tracts that controlled muscle activity, the nerve fibers, in other words, that governed voluntary movement. Any disturbance of blood supply here, even a small one, resulted in widespread paralysis, packed tightly as these fibers were. I sketched now in broad, dramatic accents, adorned with fierce lightning and ominous cloud, bleakly visualizing the cataclysm, for it was here where Mom's hypothetical crumb would have lodged.

Grey, black, and white shadows danced eerily across the screen, almost maniacally, yet with a certain order and rhythm. The nurse applied the probe to Mom's chest, her face intent yet distant. I could not fathom her thoughts, infer good or bad. There were straight and wavy lines that moved in and out, rose and fell, twittered and flittered with each beat of her heart. It was a soothing meter, a wondrous tempo resonant within her chest. It seemed never to change, a dependable cadence upon which life was based.

The lines moved fluidly, with symmetry and grace; the oscilloscope illustrating the perfect marriage of anatomy and physiology, of structure and function. The lines swelled and contracted, relaxed and braced, received and ejected, gorged and emptied. It was the sky, earth, sun, moon, day, night, yin and yang, all contained within the brittle, undulating lines of her heart - the measure of life, a microcosm of nature, the monotonous adagio of cardiac movement. Elegant, hypnotic even, but was there a thrombus?

Mom still did not stir. With the audible whir of technology around her, a nurse and son present, with the lights and sounds and slippery probe upon her chest, and no end of metaphysical flights of fancy, she remained asleep. And, so, I mused, once more, could not, in fact, think of anything else.

If this meaningless fragment had nested in a branch of the middle cerebral artery, an utterly inconsequential crumb, an insignificant speck, quartered in a vessel feeding a small segment of brain, what cascade of events would have ensued? What civil unrest in so ethereal a sphere would have arisen? I contemplated the majesty of the human brain, the domain over which it presided, and, in my mother's case, the calamity that befell it. It was an indulgence but a necessary one for I found twisted sustenance in the language of my ruminations and the labor to wrap my mind around the harsh reality of stroke.

If such a speck had settled there, in the celestial realm of the cerebral cortex, in this tangle of nerve and ganglia, where epiphanies were sounded and proclamations decreed, where sense organs delivered testimony about the world, where thought and consciousness inexplicably dwelled, where creativity stirred, where morality evolved, where philosophy took root; where the mind resided, where personality held court, where the soul sat as silent witness, and where God bestowed a small tincture of Himself – what would happen?

If such a speck took residence here and attracted platelets, red blood cells, and fibrin, the speck growing larger, filling the lumen, and occluding the vessel, bringing circulation to a halt, here, in the inner sanctum, which oversaw the workings of body and mind? Well, then, our harmless speck, became something else, indeed: a savage, a renegade, an assassin, sowing seeds of despair, driving neurons and fibers into an insufferable abyss, and, in so doing, destroying lives and dreams. Or, perhaps, it was just part of nature, random and indifferent, devoid of purpose, like a floe of ice, floating downstream.

The gray shadows appeared smooth, moved fluidly, described normal conduct and attitude of cardiac tissue. There were no disturbances or irregularities. No defects or calcifications. No turbulence or regurgitation. The contours and shadows depicted real time anatomy of a functioning heart, receiving and ejecting blood flawlessly. No vegetations, leaks, narrowings or thrombi.

"It didn't come from her heart, Dr. Moss."

"Thank you."

When she left, I sat by my mother, holding her hand. "Mom," I called out in the emptiness. No response. I placed my hands on her head and said a prayer. I kissed her, said goodbye, and returned to my office.

At home that evening, I took the full measure of all that had occurred. The implications of a severe stroke like this were clear: we were now at the earliest stages of what would be a protracted period of care and rehabilitation, culminating, quite possibly, in a nursing home. My robust and active mother may not even be able to sit up without two or three aides assisting her. I did not know this as fact, but I did not feel hopeful. Without some remarkable turn-around, every aspect of her life would be altered. The utterly mundane daily tasks of getting out of bed, brushing her teeth, taking a shower would become impossible except with intensive assistance and support. The simple pleasures that we enjoyed together, taking walks, sharing meals, chatting on the phone, would be completely out of reach.

It was painful just to think of my mother this way, to imagine her being unable to lift her left index finger, when mere days before she could walk miles without difficulty and took such pleasure in doing so. The unfairness of it was striking, too, and, yet, how many times in my career had I sat on the opposite side of the table, explaining to someone else, also unjustly robbed of good health, how these things happened. How odd now to find myself in this position and reacting as any layperson would – with bewilderment and outrage.

Outraged at whom? God? Life? The natural order of things? After all, my mother had led a relatively healthy life, did not smoke or drink, and was quite active. On the other hand, she did have mild diabetes, slightly elevated cholesterol, was overweight, and 78. Well, how am I thinking . . . that is, really, quite enough right there. But, and, yes, I am bargaining here. Still she was so active, could walk for miles and did so everyday, and had no prior history of vascular disease. Like all mothers, she worried too much about her children, often unnecessarily. Well, I could see how it could occur, but that changed nothing! I was outraged, and, on balance, coming at so inopportune a time and so unexpectedly, how could it not seem unfair?

I wondered how she would take it. Strokes were so terrible because they were so overwhelmingly debilitating and so abrupt. A stroke robbed you of your most basic capacities, your autonomy and independence. It struck at the core of who you were and what you did. Where once there was the power to act, now there was utter helplessness. What effect would this have on my self-regarding, high-strung mother? How would she respond to the reality of a disobedient and impaired body?

I had never thought much about strokes before, did not encounter them often in my practice, and rarely dealt with them. Until this. Now I had witnessed their heavy hand and the upheaval they wrought. I had now to consider the possibility that my mother could be bedridden for the rest of her life, that the prospects for meaningful recovery were poor.

And, strangely, there were no visible signs of the trauma that had taken place in the niches and crannies of her brain, no external evidence of the wound that had effaced the tissues that powered the left side of her body. It was obscured, showing itself only through its effects. The misshapen aspect of the oppressor itself remained concealed. I wondered if there were someway to loosen its grip, to restore her, to reignite the spark in those darkened recesses that dimly threatened her.

How removed it all seemed, how forlornly distant. Still I prayed for just such a regeneration, visualized just such micro-events occurring in her damaged brain, imagining the anoxic cells somehow replenished and restored, with new, sparkling blood conduits appearing, offering gifts of oxygen and glucose, nerve cells sprouting axonal shoots - tiny sprigs and tendrils that would make connections and take over the now aborted functions. How I yearned for her return to fullness.

I sat back in my favored leather chair and reminisced once more about other days, distant memories of innocence and sadness, but, also of humor and laughter, a necessary reprieve, visions of the past returning once again.

Henry Pinski was a familiar face to my brothers and me because we saw him so often. He was our family doctor, and Tuesday nights we walked down Crotona Park North, where we lived, turned left on "Dead Man's Hill" (Crotona Park East) where we used to go sleigh riding in the winter, turned right on Boston Road, past the Associated, the Gemini Dry Cleaners, Mr. Franklin's candy store, Julie's Bakery, Tony's Pizzeria, and the Dover Movie Theater. We continued under

*the "El" at 174th Street, up past Minford Place, where Nona
and Nono lived with Uncle Willy, past Hoe Avenue where
Aunt Rae and Aunt Sophie lived, to Bryant Avenue where
Doctor Pinski's office was. It was on the first floor of a five-
story apartment building, where he had a little shingle in the
window that said "Henry Pinski, M.D."*

*In those days, it was possible to walk around the Bronx
at night, although we began to hear stories of shootings and
other crimes. Mom worried about us cavorting at night by
ourselves, but when she was with us she was comfortable.
And once a week for a time, after dinner as it started getting dark, Cliff, Jerry, and I would walk with Mom to Doctor
Pinski's to get shots. "Chronic tonsilitis," Mom called it. We
were always getting sore throats.*

*We entered the waiting room, where the three of us
would play and horse around, as if we were at home, oblivious to the roomful of other patients who smiled tolerantly at
us and at Mom, who beamed back, proud of her small gaggle,
however unruly. Doctor Pinski came into the waiting room
and called for Mom who quickly gathered us up and paraded
us into his office.*

*Dr. Pinski was short, ashen, with grey balding pate and
abundant wrinkles; he wore a white coat, smiled, but maintained a grim aspect. He escorted us into his inner sanctum
(the exam room), where we were confronted by the peculiar
and nauseating smells of a medical office: the alcohol and me-
dicinal scents that always unsettled the stomach. In his office lay any number of odd and threatening instruments and
pieces of equipment including a metal "steamer" (actually,
an autoclave) that outwardly had the appearance of a toaster.
The sight of this object caused no end of dismay for us for it
was here that Dr. Pinski kept the hypodermic needles, the ultimate weapons of fear. He boiled the needles in the toaster to
sterilize them, and when he opened it, steam would hiss and
pour out of it in menacing clouds of hot, grey vapor.*

*When the steam cleared, we could see the glass syringes
and needles emerging in a pool of bubbling water. He used*

metal tongs to grasp a syringe and needle and placed them on a metal tray, making disturbing metallic sounds. Wearing rubber gloves, he attached the long, slender needle to the syringe, carefully interlocking the connecting parts. Then he took a vial with white liquid, he called it penicillin, and drew it up. We watched nervously as the thick, milky fluid filled the syringe, knowing that he was soon to inject this creamy substance into our behinds.

Jerry, because he was the oldest, went first. He pulled down his pants and bent down while Doctor Pinski wiped his rear with some alcohol. He pierced Jerry's skinny butt and injected the medicine. We watched him squirm while Doctor Pinski squeezed the syringe, pushing the white liquid in slowly because it was so thick. Because his younger brothers were watching, Jerry tried to look cool and did not cry or say a word. Then it was my turn. I bent down, felt the coolness of the alcohol on my rear, the point of the needle, and the thick medicine entering my flesh. I flinched but didn't say a word either, just like Jerry. When Dr. Pinski finished and pulled the needle out, I felt as cool as Jerry, perhaps even cooler since I was younger.

Then came Cliff, who at age three had no idea of taking pain and being cool. None of this meant anything to him, because as soon as I pulled my pants up, Cliff, understanding fully what was coming, took off like a rabbit, climbing over Doctor Pinski's desk, in front of the exam table, behind the coat rack, under the instrument stand with the needles, past the white skeleton standing in the corner, and into the bathroom where he shut the door. We ran after him and he began screaming "no, no, I don't want no shot, no, get away, leave me alone, get off of me, ahhhhh!" Mom finally grabbed him and wrestled him down into Doctor Pinski's chair, unbuckled his belt, and pulled down his pants.

Doctor Pinski smiled (stiffly) as if everything were OK and understood the little runt did not like needles. We watched him pick out another syringe from the toaster, draw up the ominous white liquid, tap the syringe to get the bub-

bles out, shoot out a fine spray from the point of the needle, doing all this in front of Cliff, who howled like a dog, squealing and crying, struggling to break free of Mom's grip. Doctor Pinski still smiled as he wiped Cliff's little behind with alcohol. Cliff continued screaming "no, no, no, I don't want no needles, Mommy, help, ahhhhh!" Jerry and I kept laughing, while Mom and now a nurse held him down. But Cliff managed to break loose and squirm to the floor, yet again, crawling under the chair.

"You gosh darn kid," Mom yelled, "geddovaheah," and she pounced on him, yanking him back up to the chair. Now, Doctor Pinski wasn't smiling.

The nurse and my mother held him against the chair, bent him down, butt out, and still he was twisting around. Doctor Pinski was trying to get a fix on him, moving his needle round and round, trying to follow Cliff's moving behind. Unable to get a bead on him, Doctor Pinski, whacked Cliff in the butt twice, "Stop it, stop it, do you hear me, stop moving!" he shouted angrily.

My mother, now furious with Doctor Pinski, yelled, "What in the hell are you doing, hittin' my kid, you've got some nerve."

"I'm sorry, Mrs. Moss, I meant nothing. It's just he's moving so much."

"I don't give a damn if he is moving," Mom shouted back, "don't ever hit my kid!" Cliff kept screaming, Jerry and I kept laughing, and Doctor Pinski finally got a bead on the target, shot straight and true, and Cliff let out a wild yelp.

Doctor Pinski injected all the medicine. Cliff was pulling up his pants, whimpering. Mom held and comforted him, and suddenly there was peace. Doctor Pinski apologized, Mom said she understood, it was OK, and by the way do you have any cough medicine for the kids, it's tough without a father. Of course, Mrs. Moss, and some candy, too, and we were on our way.

-10-

When I returned to my office the next morning, I told my secretary to call Dr. Michael Hobson, professor of Neurology at the Medical Center in Indianapolis. This was our medical Mecca, where those of us in the outback looked for guidance and advice. I frequently contacted physicians in my own field, but rarely had reason to go outside my own specialty. I sat down, thumbing through the NINDS article, published in the New England Journal of Medicine. This, of course, made it scriptural.

I had skimmed the article already, highlighting parts that seemed particularly important. I usually just looked at the abstract, then the conclusions. Who had time to go through materials, methods, and commentary? But in this case, I tarried, reading it in its entirety.

TPA or *tissue plasminogen activase* was a potent anticoagulant (blood thinner) that dissolved clots, hence the locution, "clot buster." Physicians had used it extensively for years in the treatment of heart attacks. Because of its success in treating heart attack victims, researchers then investigated its efficacy in the management of stroke. The landmark study was "NINDS." In this study, researchers found that patients receiving TPA within three hours of symptoms were 30% more likely to do well three months later than patients given placebo. But, there was a 6% increase in intracranial hemorrhage. Overall mortality, though, at three months was no different in the two groups. They concluded that despite an increased rate of intracranial hemorrhage, the use of TPA *within three hours* of symptoms did not increase mortality and improved neurologic outcome at three months.

That was it in a nutshell, and what a bombshell it had been.

The phone rang. The intercom came on: "Dr. Moss, it's Dr. Hobson."

"Hello," I said.

"Hello, Dr. Hobson speaking."

I introduced myself. "I wanted to ask you a few questions, about my mother."

"Of course."

He was pleasant enough. Most of the professors were polite when I called.

"She's 78, has some mild diabetes. She had a stroke a few days ago."

I explained to him the details, in particular, the sequence of events leading up to her arrival at the ER. "At the time no one suggested anything about TPA. I wasn't sure about the exact time of onset of the stroke. We didn't give it, and no one said much about it, but I'm wondering if we should have."

"But you weren't sure of the exact onset."

"Right, but shouldn't I have assumed it was most likely when she fell into the chair?" I asked.

"How would you know if you weren't with her?"

"But isn't the likelihood that she would have had the stroke just at that time?" I was regretting this conversation.

"Not necessarily," he said.

"You wouldn't assume that she had the stroke in the chair?"

"No, because it could have been a stroke in progress. She could have had slurred speech two hours before and still have been able to walk. You don't know unless you were actually with her. Being able to walk doesn't mean she didn't already have the stroke," he said.

"So not being with her before, there was no way of knowing when the stroke actually began?"

"Right," he said.

"And you wouldn't have given her the TPA?"

"Absolutely not. I've seen strokes evolve over days. You have to go by the last time she was definitely normal."

"Which was three hours before when I dropped her off at home."

"If that was the last time you saw her."

"She could have had the stroke at any time during that three-hour period between dropping her off and when I saw her next?"

"Right," he said.

"And you wouldn't have taken a chance with the TPA?"

"No. The inclusion criteria for TPA are strict. There is no indication for the use of TPA if more than three hours have passed from the onset of symptoms or if there's any uncertainty about when the stroke started."

"I spoke with the chairman recently," he continued. "He's reporting a twelve percent incidence of hemorrhage within three hours, not the six percent reported by NINDS. And the last thing you want with acute ischemic stroke is hemorrhage. If the initial stroke doesn't kill them the hemorrhage will. Leaky membranes and all that. I wouldn't second-guess yourself on this, Richard. TPA is a risky drug no matter when you give it and especially outside of the three hour time constraints."

"You would have been comfortable withholding the TPA?"

"Absolutely. Far more comfortable than giving it," he said.

"So TPA isn't the wonder drug with strokes that it is with heart attacks?"

"With acute MI, it's the standard of care. Not with strokes."

"Do you use the drug at all?"

"I'm very hesitant. Twenty years from now, we won't be using TPA. There'll be something much better."

"If I had given her the TPA, would it have prevented the stroke from progressing?"

"Not necessarily."

"You've seen strokes progress even after receiving TPA?"

"Yes, not to mention the risk of bleeding."

"Under the circumstances, you'd have done nothing?"

"I'd have considered her ineligible for treatment."

It was an epiphany that changed nothing, for my mother was still bedridden.

My nurse called me. I had other questions but no time. "Dr. Hobson, it's great speaking to you, very enlightening. Thanks."

I returned to the scene of the crime, which was to say my patio, carefully replaying the events as they unfolded in my memory. Unbeknownst to him, Dr. Hobson's words had greatly comforted me. I didn't think he had altered his opinions to reflect my emotional needs. Still, something in me needed to review the events before exculpating myself. I saw my mother walking out of the back door and sitting in the green lawn chair, where she always sat. It was more a vision now, vague and distant, as if glimpsed peripherally, with all movement slowed and otherworldly. Generally, she waved and said hello. This time she didn't. She sat there. But she had walked normally. I hadn't noticed anything unusual at first. Wouldn't she have said something to me? Perhaps not. Slight weakness and slurring, minor parathesias (tingling, numbness), may well have gone unnoticed by her, or, at least, not invested with great significance.

Mom was not herself in many ways anyway, being 78, very forgetful, easily confused; she had already shown early signs of dementia before the stroke. It was entirely conceivable that the initial phases of the stroke had occurred before she sat down in the chair. I told myself this (wary of possible self-serving interest), and it seemed plausible.

I had not seen her for three hours, since dropping her off from the restaurant at 3 p.m. Now it was 6 p.m. That gap was the interval unaccounted for, the unknown ellipse within which the critical event may have occurred. And there was no way to know. Was I deluding myself, rationalizing to salvage self-respect and end the self-recrimination? If what Dr. Hobson said was true, then there was no way of knowing. And a decision to administer TPA may have caused greater harm than had already beset her.

It was a beautiful day, the day of the stroke. Ying was in the house preparing dinner. Arielle and Noah were picking cherry tomatoes and green peppers from our garden. The tomatoes were ripe and full, even sweet. The kids were popping them in their mouths like candy while happily filling their buckets. It was September in every sense of the word, the summer very much with us, still effulgent and lusty, only milder and hence even more alluring.

The trees swayed boisterously in the breeze as if hearkening to the advent of autumn, but in no way reconciled to their approaching decline. Flowers bloomed, almost too beautiful to behold, so lavish was their color, scent, and texture. Flying insects pillaged them, hungrily imbibing nectar and pollen before whirring off, or, in the case of a butterfly, fluttering waywardly, as if tipsy. All the disparate elements had converged seamlessly, as if guided by some divine orchestral leader, to reach an indelible moment of perfection. Mom had tilted her head strangely. Paradise in Indiana was threatened. When did it happen? When did that final piece of debris lodge in her artery?

"Mom, are you OK?" I had asked her.

The sun had descended, producing a glorious light, golden and warm. She had made it to the green lawn chair on the patio, but when I thought back, I realized that she had not sat down as much as she had slumped down. At the time, it had not registered. I continued watching the kids, telling them to be careful, addressing them, not my mother. But little flashes were going off, tiny flares, beginning to draw my attention. Mom had not said anything, not even waved.

"Mom, are you OK?" I asked again. There was no response, but she continued looking this way. Maybe she had not heard me. I had checked her hearing last year in my office and it was good.

Could she have opened the patio door, sauntered out and sat down, even slumped down as she had, yet still under the debilitating influence of a stroke? It must have occurred then, I told myself, backsliding, ready to begin torturing myself again. But the stroke may have been "in progress," as Dr. Hobson had termed it, at least it was a consideration. The internal warfare continued. The three-hour gap. What happened that increased the risks so greatly after three hours? Leaky membranes, he had said in passing. Leaky, membranes, indeed.

Her head had an odd tilt, and she had not said a word or waved. I walked over. "Mom, are you OK?" I asked again.

"Noahcccrrr. Thaaatccchhh Noahcchhhrr." Something about Noah.

"What happened, Mom?"

"Noahcchhr, that kid, I rrccchhhannnrr." Incomprehensible. "I ran up and downrrrcchhh." She had run up and down after Noah. "I was runncchhrr up andcchhrr down the stairsccchhhrrrr. I wasccchhhrrr worried about Noahcchhrrrrr."

I ran through the events, the sudden realization that my mother was having a stroke, the call to the ER, the ambulance, the conversations with the ER physician and then Regan, and the decision to forego the TPA. And none of it mattered. The three-hour interval before I had seen her was the unknown that rendered all discussion moot. And I had asked her. "When did it start, Ma," I said, "when did you start acting this way?" But she could not answer, either because she did not know or because she could not respond. Only the gibberish about Noah. And so the conundrum remained.

I recoiled from my complacence, the ease with which I seemed willing to forgive myself, wondering if Hobson had indulged me. But that was unlikely. The discussion about three hours was probably quite legitimate. Also useful for my purposes. Which were what? To absolve myself? Would it not be better to assume that I had failed and accept the burden of my failure without the palliatives? I had not pursued arduously her defense, had not conducted myself honorably on her behalf, she who had never failed me! In my one opportunity to garner resources and act decisively, I had been found wanting, defeated by pretense and inertia. And this would remain a blight.

Comforting words by others could not relieve it. Perhaps Hobson was right that I may have incurred more harm by acting, but that did not change the *moral* verdict. Yet, even murderers were forgiven. And this did not approximate that threshold of depravity. But if there were a path to redemption, this one at least would be acceptable: to confess my guilt and be done with it. I could appeal to her directly and ask her forgiveness, but she would look at me as if I were touched. And why burden her with my guilt? In any event, she was certainly not ready for it now.

To whom could I appeal? To God? Such notions, of course, were absurd to many, especially to those who placed their faith in the temple of their squeaky little intellects. But who cared? (And what other choice did I have, for I must live!) Was it wrong for a believer (and a man of science) to come before Him, to place my sins and wretchedness before Him, so that I could do something greater than wallow in anguish? I would find a cure, some cure for her, some way to undo the harm; and if no such elixir existed, I would seek diligently all avenues of restoring her so that she could return home. Was it my fault? This question would continue to haunt me.

I looked across my desk, deluged once again by the clutter of my daily mail. Would it not be easier just to chuck it all in the garbage and spare myself the time and trouble of opening each item and *then* discarding it? I glanced at the NINDS article sitting off to the side. Dog-eared, highlighted and underlined, already worn, withered, and aged. I looked away. Pictures of my two children smiling adorably had a place on my desk. I felt a small bubble of lightness. Then another photo to the side of the others, this of my wife as a graduating nursing student receiving her diploma from the King of Thailand himself (a customary but nonetheless prized photo for all graduates in Siam).

I discarded my mail unceremoniously and returned home.

Later, I spoke with Regan. I called him at his home, late. Internists, especially this internist – talented, young, energetic – were on call twenty-four hours a day, seven days a week. Another phone call would add or detract little to the endless stream of provocations that already plagued him.

"How is she?" I asked.

"About the same, Rick." He sounded tired.

"What's the deal with the three hour time constraints?"

"You mean with TPA?" he asked.

"Yes."

"It's not recommended after three hours."

"Why?" I asked.

"Leaky membranes." That odd little phrase again.

"The mechanism?" I asked.

"Hypoxic changes – ion fluxes, free radicals. The
disruption of cell membranes."

"And then what happens?"

"The tissues become friable and the risk of bleeding goes up. Only now you've got non-clottable blood,
because you've got TPA on board. That's why we
wouldn't give it without knowing for sure you're within three hours of the stroke."

I was frustrated. At this point it was academic anyway. The critical moment for action had passed and I
was left only with the aftermath of a missed opportunity.

I returned to my texts. The huge volumes sat gravely upon several of the shelves, not like the other shelves
with the chirpy travel books. These seemed literally to
spring forth and dance. They enticed me to open and
enjoy them. Mexico. Central America. South America.
Asia. Africa. Guidebooks, well worn and used. These
were reminders of earlier years of high adventure and
exploits. They served now only to tease. There were
small figurines and other carved pieces and ceramics.
From Guatemala, Honduras, Ecuador, and Peru. I had
always wanted to take my mother on such adventures.
There was time, you always told yourself. And, suddenly, the time vanished.

I picked out an Internal Medicine tome this time.
It was not a joyful selection. Cellular death was the
topic, to understand exactly what it was that killed a
cell when you deprived it of oxygen. It was a brutal

process, I knew, on an ultramicroscopic level, and, like a voyeur, I wanted to peer in.

Noah happened to walk into the room at that moment, wanting to play.

"I will, son, in a minute."

He was cross. He had been waiting all day. He was insistent, but today he would wait. I promised him the greatest gift I could offer, which, for him, was to play baseball, but later. He was pacified, my young star, and I had my moment. The fan spun above me. The window was open. Pleasant sounds entered the room. Crickets. Birds. Children's voices. I leaned back in my chair, which squeaked slightly, and I began reading.

Oxygen was the vital fuel, the gasoline of the body and of all the tissues of the body. It was the brain that was most sensitive to its absence. Within minutes, affected brain cells underwent an irrevocable process leading to cellular death. The "leaky membranes" I kept hearing about were an end stage of the algorithm. I looked out the window. Noah was playing with a stick and smacking it against the trunk of a tree as if engaged in a battle to the death. Bits and pieces of the tree flew off, and I heard him scream proudly for Arielle to come and admire his handiwork. He was content and I was busy, and so I allowed him to continue mangling the tree. I returned to the text. Such miniscule print, not at all inviting. I continued.

The greatest works, thoughts, and writings of man, his most noble endeavors (and his most craven exploits), along with all the routine and complex faculties the brain oversaw (eating, ambulating, the vegetative functions), were founded on the process of maintaining sodium, potassium, and calcium (the "ions") in their proper compartments (within and without the cell). Absent this, nothing happened. When the ions equilibrated (within minutes of hypoxic injury), all brain function – the great, the glorious, and the mundane – promptly ceased.

It was unexpectedly bracing, almost intoxicating in its unintended vision of chaos and violence, of worlds colliding, of upheaval and convulsion unleashed within the tiny cell of the brain deprived of oxygen. On the one hand, it seemed almost trivial, the elements of such tragedy well below the threshold of normal human perception, observable only through the prism of the biochemist, whose tedious and painstaking methods measured and identified the principals in aliquots or nanograms. On the other hand, its effects on the total being, the person, were all too observable.

The final calamity was the disruption of cellular membranes (our oft-heard "leaky membranes"), brought on by the formation of free radicals, itself brought on by the presence of excess calcium within the cell, itself brought on by the failure of ion "pumps" to maintain ion "gradients," itself brought on by the lack of oxygen (etc.). The disruption of cellular membranes at some point lead to a literal bursting or rupture of the cell, which thereby ceased to exist as an entity. It had, in effect, merged with its environment, commingled and dissolved, became indistinct and inseparable, its rapid descent into oblivion complete in only minutes: a swift decline from the dizzying apogee of cellular function to that of abject and moribund disintegration reduced to a deflated lipid bag, torn and fragmented, emptied of content, of its priceless cellular machinery upon which life was built. It was tragic, in itself and in its implications.

This dissolution of the cell from a separate functioning entity to something defunct, shapeless, and indistinct from its environment carried resonances of eastern thought: the notion of our connectedness and the unity of life. The price paid to achieve this universality, though, was death: death of the self (or the cell, the single cell, as self). It was not the grand vision of the transcendent absolute parried about in religious circles, but something else, something quite tormented and deranged.

While on some level the concept worked, similarities between people, of course, abounding, yet, in many ways it was tiresome sophistry. Separateness, borders, fences, boundaries, walls, moats, gates, cellular membranes, what have you, were at least as indispensable to healthy, normal function, as our interrelatedness was. When I thought of my mother wounded as such, how I yearned for those very borders, fences, and cellular membranes that had allowed her to function fully. As for our now ruptured (enlightened?) cell – multiply this many times over, thousands, millions, or more, and you had, well, a stroke.

I gazed outside the window, a reprieve. The sun had fallen below the horizon, but there was adequate light. Parents and children still basked in the twilight. For once, I had timed it perfectly. Noah was upon me, his patience at an end. He was fiery and insistent. He demanded that I put my book down immediately and play with him. And I complied.

I put Noah and Arielle to sleep. Not, of course, before reading them a story, and then there was more, for they had become accustomed to nightly renditions of accounts about life in the Bronx. This had developed into a prominent feature of the ritual of sending them off to slumber. If I did not feel up to telling them another Bronx story, they complained bitterly. I would offer to read them a story, but that would not do. Only tales of the Bronx satisfied them – stories about their father and uncles as children, and of their Nona.

The dozens of library books I picked out each weekend sat in a corner of their room unread. And I complained to them about that. But they ignored me. These books, which formerly had satisfied them, had become quite inadequate. Stories of my travels through Asia and South America would not appease them either.

Accounts of motorcycle journeys through the Himala-
yas or wandering in the Sahara or hitchhiking around
the United States were substandard themes. Only the
red meat of the Bronx, their ancestral homeland, would
suffice, the chronicles that by now had taken on the
aura of myth, to be remembered and handed down
orally through the generations. And, so, I told them of
yet another such adventure from my past.

*Two weeks after Doctor Pinski whacked Cliff in the butt
twice, something Mom still talked about, we were on our
way to see him again. We walked down the stairs from our
apartment building and onto the street where we turned left
heading east on Crotona Park. When we arrived at the corner, we saw a crowd of people standing outside the entrance
to a building half way down the block. There were police cars
parked with flashing red lights and a wall of blue uniforms
in front of the entrance. We walked toward the crowd, curious, and when we got there, Jerry and I took off before Mom
could stop us.*

*"Hey, what are you stupid kids doing," she yelled, but
we squirmed through the throng before she could catch us.
We then muscled our way up the stairs, past a couple of blue
uniforms that didn't notice, and into the building where a
portly cop appeared.*

"Keep back, kids," he said, "you shouldn't be heah."

"What happened, officer," Jerry asked.

"Ya don't wanna know, kids."

"Yeah, but what happened anyway?" I asked.

"Pipe down, wouldja."

*I noticed a trail of blood leading up the stairs. "Wow,
what's that," I said, jabbing Jerry. "Hey, officer, what's that
blood over there?" I asked.*

"Ah, Jeez, wouldjoo kids shuddup?"

"But there's blood there," I said.

"I godda detective heah."

"Did someone get shot?" Jerry asked.

"A genius, a genius wit' a mout'."

Another cop walked over to the burly cop holding us back. "It looks like it was her husband, sir, stabbed her about a hundred times."

"Ah, Jeez, already, twenty years I never seen any ding like 'dis. Awright, bring 'er out, keep everyone back."

Two men appeared carrying a stretcher with a woman's body covered in gauze and tape from head to toe with bloodstains everywhere. Jerry whispered that it looked like a mummy. Everyone was silent, staring at the body covered in bloody gauze. One man wearing a hat took it off and held it over his chest. Some were crying, but mostly everyone gazed in horror and disbelief.

"Is she dead, officer," I asked.

"Oh, she's dead alright."

"Why, sir, why'd he do it?" I asked.

"Jeez, son, don't ask me, the whole neighborhood's gone ta hell, now run along to ya mudda."

We watched as they carried the woman's body down the stairs and through the doors of the ambulance.

"Bloody murder," Jerry called it. We ran down the stairs, through the crowd, to Mom and Cliff.

"Oh, God, kids, what happened?" Mom asked, holding us in her arms, almost crying. "Bloody murder," Jerry said. "Oh God in heaven, what's happening to the Bronx," she said, as if the Bronx were a person.

We walked to Doctor Pinski's for our shots. Cliff ran and screamed like always, shaking his chubby butt, except this time Doctor Pinski didn't smack him. Mom kept a close eye on him. We returned home to quiet streets, talking about the mummy and the night of bloody murder.

I looked at my kids, lying in bed, their eyes wide open, wondering, perhaps, from the safety of their Indiana home, what it would be like to grow up in a place like the Bronx.

-11-

I visited my mother. She was still sleeping in the telemetry unit. Still attached to the IV, the pulse oxymeter, and the EKG monitor. The room was compact, eerie and windowless. Of all things, my mother needed a view. If she were awake, she would have gone crazy in this little dungeon. Perhaps, it was better that she slept. Her face was amazingly placid, so unlike her. My mother was rarely placid. She loved nature, which often calmed her. Any variant of nature would do. Mountains, ocean, forests, meadows, and sunsets, which she loved best of all. Otherwise, a horde of loosely connected anxieties preyed upon her endlessly.

The dim lights over the head of her bed cast shadows on her face, making her appear somewhat ghoulish. Her silver hair spread regally against the pillow beneath her. She breathed deeply and hypnotically, a steady sonorous rhythm, like a chant. Her bed was her companion now, where she spent her days with strangers observing her, prodding and piercing her, drawing blood samples, analyzing her urine, monitoring her vital signs, cleansing her, perhaps speaking to her – to no avail, the shrill sounds incapable of penetrating the dense cloud that surrounded her.

I watched the lights flashing about her, from the monitor. Everything was quite adequate, the numbers satisfactory, except she remained unresponsive. The IV fluid continued dripping, a slow, soothing tempo. The bag was almost empty. As if reading my thoughts, the nurse walked in to replace it. I watched her adjust the rate, making certain the connections were good, and tracking the clear fluid as it streamed down through the catheter and into my mother's vein.

"She seems to be doing alright," she said.

I nodded.

"Does your mother live in Jasper, Dr. Moss?"

"No, she was just visiting."

"Where's she from?"

"New York."

"So she had this while she was out visiting?"

"Yeah."

"Oh, I'm sorry. How long was she here?"

"Just a week."

"Really?"

"Yeah."

"That's too bad."

So it was. A freakish thing. But the initial shock of her disease and my subsequent failures had receded. My attention now focused elsewhere, to restoring her if possible. I nodded to the nurse who left the room and returned to the ICU. I sat with Mom a while. She was stable and sleeping. I returned to the office.

Cliff called again, another annoying exercise, in the middle of a busy clinic. He was still angry, demanding explanations, as if he lived in some paradise where calamities never occurred.

"So what's up wit' Ma," he asked with an attitude.

"She's still sleeping," I said.

"Ya mean she hasn't woken up yet?"

"For a moment, here and there. Very little. She hasn't said a word."

"So whut's going on?"

"Nothing is going on," I said.

"How long is 'dis crap gonna take?"

"Days. I don't know, maybe longer."

"Isn't 'dere somethin' we can be doin'?"

"When she starts to wake up, we'll get her going with rehab and other things, but until she wakes up there's nothing we can do." I listened to him breathing.

"She's in no danger, she's OK?"

"Yeah, she's OK, vital signs are OK."

"She's still in the ICU?" he asked.

"No, she's been moved to telemetry."

"So that's a good sign?"

"Yeah, it's alright; she's still sleeping, but she's stable."

"Maybe we oughta move her?" he said.

"Where do you want to take her?

"I dunno, why does 'dis gotta happen out 'dere wit you hillbillies?"

When I got off the phone with Cliff, I called Regan.

"So what's the story with her sleeping?"

"It's that post stroke encephalopathy," he said, "they sleep for days."

"Is there anything else we can be doing?" I said, mirroring my brother's questions, which obviously had affected me.

"Not really, Rick, she's on heparin, she's being monitored, she's stable. We can't do much until she wakes up." A tinge of irritation in his voice.

"So we just have to wait?" I asked, knowing the answer.

"I'm afraid so, Rick."

My office nurse, Janet, called me to begin seeing patients. I was counting on her getting me through the day. She was glowing, fresh, and smiling. One of our first patients of the day, coincidentally, was a stroke patient from a local nursing home. He came in a wheelchair, an old man with difficulty swallowing. His wife was with him. How odd for me to see stroke patients now. I had an expanded sense of empathy with him. I felt somehow wounded in his presence, as if his disease had afflicted me. My focus on the man was pointed. I saw my mother in him. Her disease had altered my emotional range, opened up new categories of experience and sensation, even unwanted ones.

I moved slowly; I had time for my patient now. He was in surprisingly good spirits despite his dim prospects, sharply dressed, with shirt and tie, and well groomed, as if to announce that even with his condition he was still vigorous and had not given up. I admired him. The stroke had occurred several months before and had left him with right-sided weakness. He also had "Broca's" aphasia, which was intensely debilitating for him for it was difficult to form coherent sentences or even to read. He was an educated man, formerly in management in one of the local companies. I watched him struggle to produce the simplest of phrases only to give up in desperation or allow his wife to complete them. Yet, I did not feel pity for him for he seemed not to need it; he still possessed dignity and humor despite his failure in executing the most mundane tasks, to mumble even a logical word or phrase.

I was keenly mindful now more than ever of the great tribute exacted by this disease, its disability and handicap. I examined his throat and larynx. He was very cooperative. I did not detect anything. No tumors or masses and the vocal cords moved well. It was part of the disease process of stroke, the loss of the fine motor control and coordination needed to complete the routine but complex task of swallowing. I told him as much, reassuring him. I wanted to get a barium swallow to make sure he was not aspirating and then see him afterwards. His wife was happy with the report.

"He used to smoke," she said, explaining her concern about cancer.

"He's fine," I told her. "It was from the stroke, not cancer."

They were Hoosiers, friendly, solid citizens, not
demanding. The wife wheeled him out. They were in
their late seventies, married more than fifty years, and
obviously devoted. Janet assisted them to the counter
and scheduled the study.

My children visited with Ying during lunch, an unexpected surprise. Their sudden presence was always
amusing to me, so out of place was their playful banter
and antics in the austere atmosphere of a doctor's office. They burst in, laughing and loud. Noah ran to me
first, racing to make sure he arrived before Arielle.

"Hi, Daddy," he said, out of breath.

"How's everyone," I asked.

"Fine," Ying said. "He wanted to see his daddy,"
smiling and nodding toward Noah.

"Oh, you did, did you?" I said tickling him. He giggled, jumped, and overreacted. "OK, OK, calm down,"
I said. I planned to see Mom during lunch and announced my intentions, figuring this to be a good opportunity to bring the whole family to see her.

We went to the hospital and entered my mother's
room, where she remained as before. The nurse told me
she was stable, a word I was beginning to grow sick
of. The monitor showed good numbers, the beeping
sounds displaying a reassuring rhythm. The room was
dark and dismal, as always, an alien environment for
the children.

Usually rambunctious and undisciplined in public, they were uncharacteristically quiet. They stared at
their grandmother who did not recognize or acknowledge them, who continued communing only within
herself. It was odd for them to be here, I knew, but
they needed to see their Nona. I ushered them up to
her bedside. It was somber, almost sepulchral. The kids
were reticent and said hello hesitantly (at my urging),
and then they looked at each other as if they had done
something silly.

"Hold her hand and tell her you miss her." This made them feel even more foolish, but, with slight nudging, they complied. They gazed at her with puzzled looks, as if wondering why she did not awaken. They saw no visible signs of her disease, no injury or trauma to explain her inaction.

"Why is Nona sleeping," Arielle asked.

"She's sick," I said. "Remember when she had the stroke?" And they nodded. They seemed spellbound by the odd spectacle of their somnolent grandmother, she who had always been lively and vibrant, easily annoyed, yes, but loving and attentive.

"I remember" Noah said, "when she was blowing bubbles." This comment, not meant disrespectfully, was cute in a way, and referred to her difficulties in speaking he had noted, the evening of the stroke.

"Right," I said, smiling at Noah's clever depiction.

Ying bowed before my sleeping mother, Thai style, placing her pressed palms before her head, the highest point, to denote the uppermost level of respect. She told the kids to bow to Nona as well. And, so, they bid Nona farewell.

Before leaving, I checked with the nurse.

"She's OK?" I asked.

"Yes, she's stable."

"Has Dr. Regan been in to see her?"

"Yes," she said. I looked in on Mom again. Still sleeping. I could barely stand the status quo. Noah began tugging at my hand, "Come on, Daddy, let's go." We walked out. I returned to my office, Arielle to her school, and Noah and Ying back home.

My brother Jack called. I had spoken with him already and he was checking up on Mom again. That he did so was encouraging, engulfed, as he was, in a sea of personal problems.

"How's it going, Jack?" I said, breaking from a patient in order to take his call.

"So, so," he said. "How's Ma doin'?"

"Ok, nothing has changed since you called last, she's stable," I repeated the now familiar theme.

"So, she's OK?"

"Yeah, I guess," I said, his question depressing me. "Nothing really going on. Her vital signs are OK, but she's still sleeping."

The continuous sleeping was irking me; I couldn't stand talking about it.

"Does she wake up at all?" he asked.

"For a few moments, that's about it."

"She's not in a coma?"

"No, no," I said unhappily. "She responds to verbal stimuli, just tired."

"What do the doctors say?" he asked.

His questions were all acceptable, but I still resented them, pointed reminders, as they were, of my own failures. They only motivated me to find answers. I answered in a daze: "That it's normal; it'll take time."

To change the topic, I quickly asked, "So what's up with you?"

"Nothin', whaddaya want me to say, life's a bitch."

"What's going on with Rachel," I asked, inquiring about his wife.

"The same. She's in bed all day. She just got out of the hospital a couple days ago; she's depressed."

"How are the kids doing?"

"They're fine, Frank's fine, going to college, Pam's doing well in school." He suddenly sounded upbeat.

"They're OK with Rachel?"

"Yeah, they're used to it." he said.

Jack had been insecure for much of his life, brought on by a number of factors, not the least of which was a severe case of acne as a teenager. He was skinny, had terrible posture (something Mom tried passionately to correct), and intimidated no one. He became withdrawn and introspective, but read avidly and wrote for a time. He finished high school, then worked in the garment industry, which he left, finally settling on washing windows, an odd choice for someone so cerebral.

Of late, Jack had gotten into the business of selling old books, out of print, along with other collector's items and antiques, a natural outlet for him. He scoured the small towns and hamlets of upstate New York, looking for the odd bookshop or yard sale with a dusty classic or tome of some sort, autographed, perhaps, to be picked up for a pittance and sold on the internet for a hefty profit, a nice little business, and showing early signs of success. His house, though, had became a scene of great chaos, with piles of books and other clutter lying strewn about.

Yet, Jack seemed to find solace in what he did, cleaning dirty windows, transforming them into bright and transparent portals (he called his business "Bright Day"), or converting one person's discarded junk (dusty, yellowed volumes) into a prized possession for another, a kind of alchemy. Money was still a problem, as it always was. He was still prone to depression and, of late, angry outbursts, this last a peculiarity, given his lifelong diffidence.

"So you're coming out to see Mom?" I asked.

"Yes."

"Good."

I returned to my patient.

After office hours, I sat down in my chair and began to pour through an array of textbooks and articles. I also wanted to talk with Braun again, or Hobson, or someone, to find out what else could be done. I did not want to discover again that there was a treatment available that could have made a difference. Even an experimental drug would be a consideration, or a new therapy or form of rehabilitation. I would have been willing to gamble for the chance of improving her outcome.

But how to know what she needed while she continued to sleep? This was what was most disturbing about her condition. I had no idea. I felt my mother a victim of a war of attrition. Stroke, the clandestine killer, had dispatched my mother with guile and proficiency. The sense of violation was supreme.

I looked at the Buddhist painting, hanging from my wall, a serene Buddha gracefully sitting within a circle of flames. Ironic, it seemed, this gift from Nepal. I saw parallels with the Buddha's quest to end suffering and my own preoccupations. I had been a Buddhist once, delighting in its atomized analysis of life, its reductionist take on the Universe, all matter and perception broken down to its ultimate particulate nature, a subtle vibration, and, then, finally, nothing.

I had spent time in a Buddhist monastery, a forest temple in southern Thailand, watching the in-breath and out-breath, standard Vipassanna (inward or "insight") meditation, looking for intuitive wisdom that would deliver me from ignorance, a Buddhist form of redemption. I had decided years ago that enlightenment was unattainable and switched paths, becoming, once more, a Jew, a born-again Jew. For Mom's purposes, the Jewish path to healing and redemption seemed right: to ask the Creator for help. That of course required faith, a rare commodity.

The fluorescent light above my office desk was out. I would ask Linda to call maintenance. I looked out my window, a slender blade of a window, not unlike my mother's room, although not quite as forlorn. There was still ample light out, the equinox not quite upon us, days still longer than nights. Thus far, the stroke had been a struggle for me, although I refused to recede to my previous spells. What mattered was to remain vigilant, to avoid complacency, and to not let another opportunity slip by. I was on a hunt, my own quest for a cure, like the Buddha.

When I checked my mailbox in the hospital, there was an article from the librarian on "rehabilitative pharmacology." ". . . A new frontier . . ." it said, in the abstract. Pharmacologic intervention in the sub acute stage, *days to weeks post stroke*. I liked it. To create treatment options *after* an established stroke, after the irreversible damage had occurred. The whole emphasis on TPA, which had made such a splash in the media and the medical world, was misguided because of the need to begin treatment within three hours of the stroke, a difficult requirement to meet. This constraint, indeed, had plunged me into my own personal crisis. The number of patients that could actually be treated was very small, because most patients did not make it into the emergency rooms quickly enough.

I went to the doctor's lounge next to the radiology department to glance at the article. The lounge was a carpeted, quiet room with a computer, phone, TV, and refrigerator. It was late, so no one else was there. I sat down in one of the cushioned chairs with a bottle of carbonated water. The photos of the previous chiefs of medical staff at the hospital hung in chronologic order on the walls, a form of tribute for undertaking that difficult position with its endless stream of headaches.

I read the article. What I liked about it was the notion that one could treat patients without worrying about the hysterical three hour "window of opportunity" that was all the rage now. Emergency rooms throughout the land had adopted "protocols" for the treatment of stroke patients or "brain attacks," based on TPA and this three-hour business; less than one percent of the patients were even eligible, not to mention the potential risks. In a way it was futile, another mindless fad that had overtaken the medical world that in reality held little hope for improving outcomes for all but a tiny number of stroke victims. I took a sip from my bottle of water.

The authors were expounding on the benefits of amphetamine for enhancing recovery in the stroke survivor, wisely noting the "time constraints of the therapeutic window" of TPA. Researchers had developed dozens of such agents, as they laboriously hunted for the next miracle drug, but none was clinically useful, and all for the same reason. Everything about this article resonated with me. I wished I had seen it a few days before, when I was in crisis mode.

Animal experiments had shown improved motor recovery after unilateral ablation of the motor cortex in those animals receiving amphetamine, as long as the animals were also properly exercised (walking across a beam). The proposed mechanism was an increase in norepinephrine levels in the brain. Why would that help? The theories were interesting, almost Aquarian. They dealt with such notions as the natural "plasticity" of the brain, the ability of the damaged brain to repair or remodel itself, the unmasking of dormant connections, "redundancy," they called it, which allowed for recruitment of parallel neural pathways to take over lost functions. Then something about "diaschisis."

I looked up at the ceiling, a series of rectangular beige Styrofoam panels. Monotonous. I closed my eyes and rubbed my face. This article excited me. But it was experimental, with no randomized, controlled, clinical studies to support it. So of what use was it? Perhaps, none. The article was more an exhortation to other colleagues in the neurological community that had been chasing butterflies and impractical solutions, to look elsewhere, or, perhaps, to change the whole paradigm. I heard padded footsteps on the carpeted floor. A white coat flashed by, mumbling some sort of greeting, and then hurried out the door. One of the internists, harried as always, running off in the general direction of the ICU, where they spent much of their waking hours. I glanced at the article again, this work out of Canada.

My beeper went off. I looked at the little display. Relieved, because it showed my home phone and not the emergency room. I was needed there, a dining emergency, perhaps, or, else, my kids wanted someone to play with.

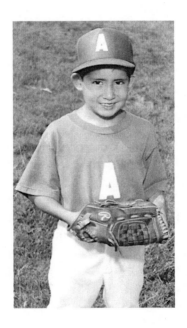

-12-

When I got home, there was a plate of steamed rice on the table, topped with cashews and vegetables sautéed in sesame oil, a glass of wine, and a salad with oil and vinegar dressing. Ying received me with a kiss.

The kids heard me walk in and ran down from the TV room, hurriedly shutting off the TV as soon as they detected the familiar sounds of my entrance, an ongoing game they played with Dad, whom they knew despised television. Noah bounded down the stairs, jumped from the first landing to the floor, fell and banged into the door of the bathroom, picked himself up unhurt, ran into the kitchen, and without any reduction in velocity, hurled himself at me like a missile, thrusting his head into my abdomen (even as I sat), which I had tensed in preparation for the impact.

"Hi, Daddy," he said, breathlessly. Arielle followed in her manner, the antipode of her younger rival, but equally effective in securing my attention. She coyly insinuated herself between me and my food.

"Hi, Dad," she said, offering me the back of her head for a fatherly kiss. Noah then decided he too needed one of my laps, and so now my children occupied both laps, which was typical; I had to navigate between the two of them and my plate of food.

"Kids," I said, "do you mind sitting next to me on the chairs so I can relax and enjoy my meal."

"No," said Noah, "I want to sit on your lap."

Ying offered assistance. "Noah, sit next to Mommy, let Daddy relax."

This offer he accepted; Arielle then moved to an adjoining seat, thus liberating my two laps and arms.

"Arielle is finishing Book Two," Ying said, referring to her violin lessons. This little process had not been easy. Arielle had started at age three, the youngest student in the local Suzuki chapter, and it had been a challenge getting her to play. Bribery (using generally, candy, chocolate, or jelly beans) was required, but after much gentle persuasion, she was becoming a respectable little violinist. She had played for Mom just before the stroke, and my mother was enchanted, for none of her own children had taken up an instrument, mainly because we could scarcely afford it.

"Congratulations," I said, beaming at my six year old.

She smiled coyly, turning her head at an angle and looking down, avoiding my eyes but still delighting in the attention. I beckoned for her and placed a fatherly pat on her head. This elicited a storm of protest from Noah, who whined and furled his brow, expressing profound displeasure at the wave of attention being lavished upon his sister. I appeased him with appropriate sounds of encouragement.

"I hear you're almost done with your 'Twinkles,'" I said, referring to the first five songs in Book One, simple tunes for beginning violinists. He smiled happily, pacified by this brief coil of parental affection.

I returned to my meal.

Later, I received a phone call from Jason Braun. "Rick, how are you," he said.

"Fine," I answered.

"I went by to see your mother and she is stable, but I'm afraid she is pretty dense."

"When will she wake up?"

"Soon, I think."

"So, you can't say much about her recovery?" I asked.

"I'm afraid not."

"What can you tell me about 'diaschisis'?"

"Diaschisis? It is an old concept. Where did you come across that?"

"In an article about post-stroke pharmacology. They mentioned the use of amphetamine; that this somehow prevented *diaschisis,* which may improve outcomes."

"Diaschisis is the process whereby damage in one area of the brain may induce damage in other distant areas of the brain that are functionally related."

"The article highlighted diaschisis as an explanation for enhanced recovery seen with the use of amphetamine."

"Yes, but it is very controversial, and unproven."

"I understand," I said.

"It is experimental, Rick; we still don't know how to improve recovery beyond the usual forms of treatment."

"But if there's something out there —"

"Of course," he said. "We will watch her and consider all options."

"I spoke to Michael Hobson," I said.

"Who?"

"At the Med Center."

"Oh. Anything useful?"

"We talked about TPA. He did not disagree with the decision not to use it." I said. I rubbed my face and eyes. "Too risky. And there is the three-hour cut-off. You know, the leaky membranes, hemorrhage, and all that."

I breathed heavily into the phone, feeling oddly reptilian. I noticed my hand quivering. What was wrong with me? I turned to find Ying staring at me. She looked aghast, as if I were on the verge of something unforgivable. "I'm gonna go and have a catch with my son," I mumbled into the phone.

"What?"

"What time is it?" I said, as if another person were speaking.

"About 7:15. Are you OK, Rick?"

"Yeah." And I laughed. And he laughed.

"I hope you are OK – *and* your mother. I will be in to see her tomorrow. Maybe she will wake up soon." Ying was still staring at me, worried.

"Thanks, Jason."

"What's the matter with you," Ying said, as I hung up.

"Where's Noah. I want to have a catch."

Why I wanted to have a catch with Noah at that moment made a great deal of sense to me. I was irrational. And I did not care.

"Noah," I yelled. I heard the little steps. Down the stairs. The wild leap from the first landing and the crash into the bathroom door. "Let's have a catch."

"Ok, Daddy."

My son was beautiful, and I loved to watch him play. He was a switch-hitter, another Mickey Mantle, I told myself, with a balanced, fluid swing that had to be a gift from God. Since age two. I did not have to teach him a thing. He was welded perfectly, his movements refined and liquid, from the very first time I had given him a plastic bat and Whiffle Ball. I will mold this one, I thought to myself.

"Throw, Daddy," he yelled. And what an arm. A southpaw. Always at the letters. Hard and tight, like he'd been playing for years. He gripped the ball and flung it, like a spear, stepping with his right foot, pivoting at the hip, the ball rolling off his outstretched fingers, as it whirled, spun, and sailed through the air, smacking the pocket of my glove with that deep, rich, satisfying *thwack*. Each time, *thwack*. What consistency! What unalloyed delight!

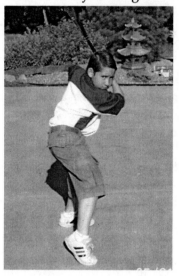

"Here's a high pop-up, son." He measured and tracked the white ball as it rose first and then fell, following its descent, circling under it, the ball accelerating, getting larger, he getting under it and - *making* the play. "Good catch, son." Field, throw, and hit, a father's dream.

And there was peace. A white, spongy T-ball with a smiley on it, a mitt (a gift from his Uncle Jerry, also a lefty), and a three-year-old boy. The evening moved fast toward night, the sky beginning its initial approaches into inky blackness, the earliest, brightest stars just appearing, the orange sun receding into a forest of purple and crimson, the temperature cooling, the air fresh, the waterfall and pond with the Koi fish gurgling, the grassy lawn resplendent and lush. And there *was* peace in the house, my mother and her disease momentarily absent from my thoughts.

I returned to my study, to my madness. I pursued with ardor my mother's cure and my cure.

I turned through the pages, the corrupted old book, dense and annotated, smudged, penciled, vile, gnarled, like an encrusted barnacle, yet possessed of a kind of truth. I perused the material already covered; saw where I had left off. The topic was *infarct*, the word itself thuggish and crude. I caressed the pages, gathering them up as if something precious. How many hours did someone spend at some benighted desk putting all this together? The lunacies that propelled men forward. The vanities and passions that tormented us. For what? More insanity. Or to create order from the harried, anarchic universe. To see the invisible designs behind the coarse manifestations; to divine divinity. Or to explain, in this case, the pathophysiology of a disease process.

I turned the pages, my scriptures, the sacred language of science.

Infarct was the outcome of an interruption in blood supply; I read hungrily, the technical language somehow soothing. A masochistic strain, perhaps? I should find it harsh and grating, as it was intended to be, but I enjoyed it instead, almost as a form of prayer, an indirect obeisance to the Almighty, who underwrote the entire enterprise in the first place. I continued.

Blood supply was everything, carrying oxygen and glucose upon which the brain depended. Its absence (a mere five minutes) triggered a sequence of events that led to cellular death and necrosis, or infarction, which was irreversible. Infarcted brain tissue was dead tissue. It softened, then liquefied. In time, a cavity formed when the dead tissue was cleared (macrophages, and the like), leaving a hole. A hole! Emptiness. A shredding of the historical record. A cavern, where once stood millions of neurons. From these neurons, songs were once sung and hands held. Toes, legs, arms, and fingers moved according to their dictates. And now, in their place, a void, a barren hollow in a sea of tangled circuitry. A defilement.

I looked outside. It was dark. Street lamps turned on. There was peace here in my little corner of the universe, yet I felt no satisfaction. I returned to my deceased neurons, and read on.

This confluence of neurons known as the brain, its trillions of cells, huffing, heaving, crackling, and wheezing, was the theater upon which the dramas and conspiracies of life were conceived. It was here where the orchestra of neural mechanisms were arrayed, organized, and integrated. It was here where data was received, processed, and interpreted, transformed, finally, into intelligence, or, at least, meaningful information. This intelligence then organized itself through ancient (neural) pathways, attaining, finally, a critical threshold of coherence that evolved into a mélange of perception, memory, and sensation, distilled yet further into the extraordinary macro-development known as consciousness.

This mystical intelligence, released, as it was, at the end of each nerve fiber, the *synapse* (or, shall we say, millions upon millions of synapses) between nerve and nerve, and nerve and muscle, the *neuromuscular junction*, conveyed through the medium of tiny packets of *acetylcholine* (a "chemical mediator"), also made possible the ballet of exquisite, tightly controlled muscular contractions (and relaxations) that resulted in . . . *movement*, and, therefore, function. This, of course, enabled us to live and create.

But, the hole! The accursed abyss. The odious graveyard of nerve tissue and axon, lying strewn and scattered like so many corpses.

And in my mother's case, I did not know the size of the "hole," how much damage was done, nor how much function would return. Nor could she tell us. She continued to sleep.

Another sleepy figure appeared at my door. This, my daughter, standing before me in pajamas, about to go to bed. "What are you doing, Daddy?" she asked, looking at me as if I were daft.

"Oh, I'm reading, honey."

"About what?"

"About strokes," I said, relaxing in her mini-presence.

"What about them?" she asked, somewhat precociously, I thought.

"Well, a stroke causes a hole," I said, finding convenient use for this metaphor.

"A hole in the head?"

"Well, in the brain."

"A big hole?" she asked.

"No, a small one, but big enough."

"Is that why Nona can't move?"

"Yes, sweetheart. Because holes can't do anything. They're just empty. So the brain can't work."

"How long has Nona been sick?" she asked.

"About six days."

"Is she going to get better?"

"It'll take time," I said.

"But she will be OK, right Daddy?"

"Yes, honey," I said more optimistically than I felt.

I kissed her and she went upstairs. I listened for her footsteps and the sound of her door closing. Then I returned to my obsessions.

I remembered the article I had read earlier, about the "plasticity" of the brain, its ability to remodel and restore itself, to recreate lost function using alternative pathways, neural sprouting, fresh connections - and limiting the damage of diaschisis. Such a word! But a valid and comprehensible concept. Limit the damage to distant but neurally related structures. Amphetamine was experimental and was therefore not available for clinical use. But was there something else? Something not conjectural; something, at least, being *used* in medical centers, and showing promise – in research protocols somewhere; something beyond the usual prescriptions, the rehab, the blood thinners, the long deserts of time spent waiting.

I glanced around the room and noticed the tapestry of fruit hanging on the wall over my desk. Soft, soothing colors, golden and brown on a background of black, muted, yet transporting. I had heard tapestries described once as "woven frescoes," the art form of Popes and Kings wishing to proclaim their power, influence, and wealth. This one was not so extravagant, nor was it, however, a mere ornament. Mom had bought it for me from an Ecuadorian employee at one of the garment factories she had worked at years ago, the effort, no doubt, of a skilled Andean weaver laboring diligently over a loom for months. She thought it was beautiful, and I agreed, promptly framing and hanging it on the wall. How excited she had been upon seeing it there the first time.

I walked into the living room where Ying, unexpectedly, was waiting. I sat with her, saying nothing of the events of this morning or of the phone call with Braun. Or of my studies and readings. I didn't want to talk, only to sit. She was agreeable. She would not force anything. She offered instead green tea, fragrant and warm, she now convinced of the health benefits of this beverage, a preventative, she insisted, loaded with antioxidants. I sipped it. It was good. Everything seemed to be conspiring against me, yet I felt relaxed. I had no further battles for the day. I looked at Ying, smiled, and I reminisced.

There was a pretty Puerto Rican girl, about 17, named Linda, who lived in our building in the Bronx with her family. All of us liked her. She had black hair, thin legs, and dimples, and spoke English with a Spanish accent.

Whenever she saw Mom, she said, "Hello, Meesus Moss," with her funny accent, "how are you?" and helped Mom if she was carrying anything. She lived on the first floor; we lived on the third floor, right by the stairs as you walked up. We ran into her every day and after Mom got to know her, she let Linda baby-sit for Cliff and me if she had to run errands. Cliff and I liked Linda and asked Mom if we could play in her house. I could tell Mom wasn't sure, but after a while relented.

We knocked on her door that first time. Linda answered, smiled, and said, "Oh, my leetle friends, come een, come een."

Her apartment was crowded with people and kids, everyone was speaking Spanish, and there was loud Spanish music coming from a radio in one of the rooms. There were pleasant aromas coming from the kitchen, where her mother (short, chubby, and aproned) was cooking. Linda introduced us to her mother, who pinched our cheeks, and said, "Que lindo!" ("How precious"). She was making pork and rice ("arroz con cerdo"). She offered us some. When Linda told me it was pork, I said, "No thank you," because Mom told us never to eat pork.

We walked into the living room, where some guys were sitting on the floor watching the Yankees – Los Jonkees, they called them – on a tiny black and white TV, smoking cigarettes and drinking beer. They were laughing, talking, sometimes yelling in Spanish at the TV. One of them looked at us and smiled, showing all of his teeth. He held up his beer can and said, "Quieres, amigos?" I looked at Cliff.

"No thanks."

"Ramon," she hissed, and smacked him on the shoulder.

"Sorry little sister, just keeding," Ramon said laughing, returning to the game.

I also saw a picture of a guy on a wall with vines wrapped around his head and rays of light shooting out from all over his body, struggling to carry some wood. There were other pictures of him riding a donkey or talking to some people at a long table during supper. They were hanging on the wall and on tables in all of the rooms and I wondered who he was.

"Dat ees Jesus," Linda told me.

"Who's he?"

"He ees God," she said.

"Huh! How could he be God?" I asked.

"Dat ees heem, Ricky."

"How do you know what God looks like?"

"We know from dee Bible."

"I never saw no picture of God before," I said.

"No?"

"He's in heaven, how can you make a picture of God? My mother has lots of picture books on the Bible, but I never saw no picture of God! An' he's not a man anyway, he's God!"

She took me over to a plastic model of the same guy stuck on some kind of cross with spikes going through his hands and feet, and those sharp thorny vines digging into his head, his eyes looking up, and red blood dripping everywhere.

"What happened to him?" I asked.

"Dees is the crucifixion."

"What?"

"The crucifixion of Christ."

"Who did that to him?"

"Dee Jews," she said.

"Huh?"

"Yes, Ricky."

"Why'd they do that?"

"They deed not understand him."

"So they killed him?"

"Yes, Ricky."

"So, how'd he get to be God?"

"Jeesus Christ, our lord and savior, is dee Son of God. He was sent by dee heavenly father to die for our sins."

Later, I spoke with my mother. "Hey, Ma, you know anything about Jesus," I asked.

"Why, who told you about Jesus?" Mom asked with a tinge of emotion in her voice.

"Linda."

"I knew I shouldn't have let you go down there."

"Did the Jews kill Jesus?"

"No, we didn't," Mom said, annoyed.

"How come Linda said we did?"

"Lies. They got nothin' better to do than lie about the Jews, like they haven't caused us enough trouble all these years. And don't you listen to a word of it, you hear me?"

"Was Jesus a Jew?"

"*Yes.*"

"*Why don't we believe in him?*"

"*We're Jews, that's why.*"

"*Why do the Puerto Ricans believe in him?*"

"*They're Catholics.*"

"*The Catholics believe in a Jew and we don't?*"

"*That's right, we just believe in God.*"

"*Is Jesus the Messiah?*"

"*No, he's not! The Messiah hasn't come yet,*" said Mom.

"*When is he coming?*"

"*We don't know, but we keep praying. In the meantime, be a good Jew and stop talking to Linda about Jesus.*"

So we stopped going down to Linda's house and Mom didn't let her baby-sit for us anymore.

A few weeks later, I was playing in the courtyard outside our building with Cliff. After a while, we got hungry and went back upstairs. One of the windowpanes in the entrance door was missing. When I put my hand on the door to open it, I felt a sharp pain and recoiled. I drew my hand back quickly and saw a stream of blood pouring from a gash in the center of my palm. I looked up and saw a small triangular piece of glass sticking out from the window frame. I pressed my hand against my stomach and yelled for Mom, crying hysterically. Just then, Linda came running down the stairs. "*Ok, niño,*" I heard her say in a comforting voice. She carried me upstairs.

Mom rushed me to the bathroom, put my hand under the faucet, and ran the cold water over it. She wrapped a towel around it tightly to stop the bleeding. Linda held the towel as Mom embraced me. She rocked and kissed me.

We sat there. Mom was singing quietly to me. Linda held my left hand, her eyes closed, as if she was praying. I calmed down. I even felt happy. A while later, Linda unwrapped the towel to look at my hand. There was a gash with yellow strands of fat and other strange particles coming out of it; but the bleeding had stopped. Mom grabbed a bottle of Mercurochrome from the cabinet.

"It won't hurt, Ricky," she said, touching the cut with the glass dropper. The orange color spread through the lines of my hand, staining the skin. Then Linda placed a bandage around it.

"How did this happen?" Mom asked.

"It was dee broken windows downstairs, Mrs. Moss."

"Goodfornothin' landlord."

"He ees slow to feex things."

"He's busy countin' his money."

"I will tell dee super."

"I'll tell him myself when I wring his Irish neck."

"Yes, Mrs. Moss."

"Thank you so much, Linda, can I give you something," Mom said.

"No, no, I am happy to help your son, Mrs. Moss. I deenk he ees OK now."

Now we could play with Linda again. Mom didn't seem to mind. We went to her apartment and stayed with her family, and the guys drinking beer, smoking cigarettes and watching Los Jonkees on TV, listening to loud Spanish music, and the beans, rice, fried fish, and barbecued pork (which we didn't eat), and all the pictures of Jesus. It was handy for Mom who had a household to run, plus work, and needed help sometimes. Linda would keep us for an afternoon and drop us off before dinner. But we played all afternoon with Linda and her family, and Mom didn't seem to mind.

-13-

I visited my mother at the hospital. She could not be aroused. I called out her name, and she opened her eyes just briefly before returning to sleep. This in itself was a revelation: the fluttering of her eyelids, the separation of the folds, the roving dark eyes in a sea of white. They appeared glazed, a thin film of mucus covering them; they moved around randomly, as if disoriented or under the influence of a dream. For a single instant, she fixed her eyes upon me.

At that point, there may have been a thin thread connecting us that promptly vanished. Whether she rose to the level of actual recognition, I did not know. Indeed, whether she had had any meaningful mental activity since the stroke, I could not say, so complete was the depth of her slumber.

Mom's eyes drifted upward and the vast gates of her eyelids slowly closed, meeting with a thud (it seemed), and separated me from her again. Her face was tranquil, unfazed by the horrendous tragedy that had befallen her. Her lips were parted as if to speak, but she uttered no words; they were pink and smooth, covered with a layer of Vaseline, applied by the nurse at my request.

I gazed at the monitor just above her bed, her constant companion, and the numbers were good: her pulse strong and steady, her oxygen levels well above 90%. Dr. Regan had restarted her heparin drip. He had stopped it, temporarily, when the stroke progressed, concerned about an intracerebral bleed. The CAT scan he had ordered, however, was negative. Her PTT (a clotting study) was 'therapeutic' when the stroke worsened, he had mentioned at the time, implying that she should have been OK. Only she wasn't. Her blood, although properly "thinned" was still viscous enough for the thrombus to propagate and move her from the benign course of a light stroke to the incivility of a dense one.

"Do you think we'll get much return," I had asked absent mindedly, forgetting that I had asked him the same question yesterday.

"I don't know, Rick." He had said slowly, as if pondering deep thoughts. "She's still pretty dense." The words had fallen from his mouth like lead pellets, crashing upon the floor. Unwanted and fractious words. But he was earnest and concerned. I knew he had another twenty or so patients scattered about the hospital in varying degrees of ill health, each with anxious loved ones, and that for him my mother's illness was not that unusual.

Since it was a holiday, I had my kids with me. They walked gingerly into the room, fascinated by the lights and sounds, quieted by the strangeness of it, to gaze upon their Nona. Two tiny innocents, generally immersed in their busy, little worlds of play and mischief, utterly indulged in a way we never were as kids, suddenly plunged into this dark mortuary of a room, the aura of illness palpable, even the aura of death. I wondered how their little minds averaged these variables, for this did not compare favorably with their usual milieu. It was all so *clinical,* and, hence, utterly foreign and indigestible. Or perhaps not. For they were hushed and silent as they entered and revealed an instinctive respect for the gravity of the moment and for their grandmother now stricken.

I tried again to wake Mom, to see if the presence of the kids would arouse her, their youthful energies somehow penetrating the thick vapors that surrounded her.

"Hold Nona's hand," I told them, and they complied, each grasping her hand and holding it, as if delivering a sacred spark. "Speak to Nona," I said.

They looked at me quizzically. Then Noah said timidly, "Hi, Nona."

"Good, son, talk to her. Tell her what we're doing today."

He nodded. "Yeah, Nona," he said, "we're gonna go swimming and take a bike ride. Then we're gonna get some food. Can you come?"

And with this, amazingly, Mom's eyelids began to flutter, parted slightly, revealing two irises, this time possessed of some measure of awareness. She looked around initially, as if an alien unaccustomed to the sight of human beings, and then gazed upon the two creatures with high-pitched voices that had summoned her. They looked back, encouraging her with their eyes to return to the world she had forsaken. For the briefest of instants, a slight smile creased her wrinkled face, registering delight at the sight of the two small faces before her. The spell quickly subsided, however, Mom's eyes receding as she returned to her echoes and dreams. I almost chuckled at my children, touched by their reverence.

"You see, kids," I said, "Nona hears you." I smiled at them, and they basked happily in the glow of their father's deep appreciation.

Just then, as if to reinstate proper perspective, the ICU nurse walked in. "That's been about it, Dr. Moss," she said, "pretty much sleeping all the time." I, however, had not seen my mother open her eyes in a week and was elated. She adjusted Mom's IV. "She seems to be waking up a little more though."

"Nothing with her left side?" I mumbled, suddenly deflated.

"No, nothing, no movement at all." She shook her head, drawing up the corner of her mouth to evince sympathy.

"She's moving the right side though," I noted.

"Yeah, when she's awake, which isn't much," she said.

"Vital signs are OK?" I said, reciting the liturgy.

"Yeah, she's stable."

I nodded and said no more. The clinical course here was torpid, almost Paleozoic: an infinitesimal progression measured in eons, it seemed. The fluttering of her eyelids and hint of a smile were reason, I felt, for joy, a great hurdle overcome, a harbinger of incredible developments to come. And, quickly, I realized, as I measured my thoughts against the reality of my mother's condition, how despondent I was. Such exaggerated euphoria for a flutter of eyelids! But, then, as if by Providence, I was rescued from despair by the shifting of my two companions, who began making irritating noises to indicate their impatience.

It was a beautiful day, a perfect day in September, a gentle month, a grand month. And I had the day off with them, my able and happy mates. I recalled how much I wanted to enjoy this perfect month with my mother. Once more, I felt the edges of regret encroaching, but the nagging of my children promptly banished further such futile yearnings. We left the unhappy room to sample the pleasures of the day, a wonderfully sunny day, as my dear mother vegetated in her little cell. Mercifully, she was oblivious, for this was her kind of day.

We rode our bikes to a nearby park, one of many in this little town. I had always felt such a bond with my mother, a sense of protectiveness for her, a role reversal that made sense in the context of our lives. By extrapolation, I had extended that understanding and experience of the mother-son relationship to all mothers and sons, endowing it with a sanctity that transcended, I felt, all other relationships. As the son of my mother, I reflected on this attachment, its nature and essence, and wondered what it was exactly that bound me to her.

I looked around at the kids. They had taken up with two other children and were running hysterically up the ladders and through the tubes and tunnels, to be vomited out some other end. They were fully content and desiring nothing else, even had I the power to grant them any wish. Fully engaged as such, no distracting thoughts befell them; their rubbery faces grinned wildly and with much brilliance, as they scurried and frolicked . . . and left me alone.

Who did not love their mother, I thought. It would take an unrepentant fool, a brute, or numbskull. Relationships, including mother and child, could become complex, but there were few among us for whom our mothers would not arouse a profound sense of allegiance and affection. After all, what could match its power and resonance? She, the giver of life, the nurturer and protector who had raised us.

But more specifically, what was the nature of the bond between my mother and me, this old woman, lying sick in her hospital bed, whom I had not lived with for twenty-five years, and now saw only once or twice a year? What was the force behind the emotions I now felt when visiting her bedside? And what was there about mother and son that was distinct and drove such force of emotion? Did this bond possess some unique property, a more pure distillation of an already consecrated link that distinguished it from other ties?

The children had shifted to the swings. These were the long-chained assemblages that could soar, the seats a mere rubber slab and unguarded. I had taught them to pump themselves, which they did, and they were already gliding at a good clip and still rising. They were laughing, shouting, and engaged.

Did this mother-son bond occupy some elevated perch; confer upon its constituents a certain sanctity? Did it bequeath a nutritive membrane that protected one, allowed one to flourish and grow, as if in a kind of greenhouse? So it seemed with my mother, who had always sustained me, her instincts generally sound and good. It was a kind of envelope, a sanctuary, and a platform from which one launched oneself into ever ascending trajectories. It was the soil to which one was rooted and from which one grew. It was an elixir, an essence that graced one with a touch of divinity, mother as Creator, who bestowed a hallowed life-giving spark.

I studied the cloud formations above, even as I listened for my children, my own parental instincts engaged, as my mother's had been through the years. They were puffy, white cumulus clouds, braced against a sea of deep blue, so luminous and stark as to be perfect, the sky now a wondrous curtain drawn across the heavens. I felt quite serene and whispered a verse from a psalm: "How lovely are Your courts, O Lord!"

Mother brought one into the world, gave life to one, and was, therefore, God-like, endowed with the power of creation. God worked through mother, preserving the promise of life. Mother, in the act of creation, became divine, and, so, invested in one the essence of divinity. I paid homage to mothers, for it was they who, after conception, were charged with the task of carrying the promise, the fertilized seed, to fruition, and endured the pain of labor before yielding to the world new life.

Mother was the earth, water, and sun, source of nourishment, giver of life, upon whom one depended for everything. Son was the promise to be fulfilled, the seedling upon whom love and affection was lavished, the avatar, the word made flesh, the embodiment of one's greatest hopes. The contours changed, the lines blurred, but the sinew and substance of it remained the same, unto death. The son was the promise waiting to be fulfilled. And the mother-son relationship was the soil within which the promise took root.

My six-year-old daughter appeared before me, she who referred to me as her "partner," and I chuckled at the sight of her. She was sweaty and warm, her hair tussled and moist from her activities. She was thirsty. She looked at me expectantly. Was I not the earth, water, and sun for her? And, then, too, for my son, who was scurrying quickly behind her. I did not ask, but imagined I knew the answer. The father deity, the sky, wind, and thunder, was also quite seminal and could be the radiant sun around which his children orbited as my mother was for me.

I walked her to the water fountain and lifted her up so she could drink, holding her against my waist with one hand and turning the water on with the other, balancing her carefully as my left arm braced her. I raised my knee up under her, managing to avoid the stream of water as it squirted out in a pleasing arc. Thirsty, she drank, taking her time, as if poised on an inert pedestal. Then she looked up at me momentarily, checking her inert pedestal, and turned to imbibe some more. She satisfied herself and ran off to join Noah.

At some point, the son became protector. Mother, source of all joy and sustenance needed help, no, needed protection, a kind of tribal reflex. Mother was sick, and I was her physician son. And I would help her, help the one who had done all in her power to shield me (and my brothers) all those years. I remember . . .

Nothing special happened between Linda, our babysitter, and us for a couple of months. She still babysat us, and Mom let us stay at her house.

One afternoon we were playing "slug" outside the house. I did not know if anyone played slug outside the Bronx, but inside the Bronx, it was a major sport. Slug was like handball but instead of hitting the ball against the wall on a fly, you hit the wall on a bounce. And usually the wall was the side of an apartment building. You used a rubber Spaulding ball instead of a little hard black ball, and the concrete squares marked off on the street were the boundaries.

We were playing slug against the wall of the red brick building next to our house, where Larry's friend, Gary lived. We played right under the windows of an older couple who lived on the first floor. They didn't like us playing there; they didn't like the yelling and arguing or the ball hitting their window. They spoke Yiddish, and the old man wore a yarmulke. When he got angry, he would shake his fist at us. Sometimes, he would pour water on us.

Cliff and I and a couple of friends from up the block were playing. One was a kid we called "Eggy," age 6, whose head was shaped like an egg; the other was "Albie" for Alberto, a Puerto Rican kid from up the block. During the game, I noticed a group of Puerto Ricans walking out of my building. I recognized some of them from Linda's family. Many of them were crying. Linda's Mom was crying worst of all, her eyes bloodshot and swollen. She could hardly walk and her children had to support her.

They walked past us, as we stood silently watching, our intense little game of slug suspended. Albie knew Spanish. He could hear some of them speaking as they passed. His eyes widened. "Ohmigod," he shouted to the rest of us.

"What?"

"Linda's been shot!"

"Get outta here!" I exclaimed.

"Somebody shot her!"

"You're crazy!"

"No, man, that's why they're cryin'."

"Where?"

"At the cleaners, where she worked!"

I took Cliff upstairs. *"What happened, Ricky,"* Mom asked, seeing me out of breath.

"Linda's been shot!" I yelled.

"What!" she screamed. *"Who told you?"*

"Albie."

"When?"

"Just now."

"Oh, God in heaven! What's going on in this stinkin' neighborhood!"

I ran down the block with Eggy and Albie, turned left on Crotona Park East, onto Boston Road, and over to the Gemini cleaners. There was a big crowd with police cars, red lights, barricades, and lots of blue uniforms. We sneaked through the crowd to the line of police standing in front of the cleaners. I could see a pair of skinny legs with black shoes lying over the doorway. I remembered those legs and shoes.

A black cop was standing in front of us. When he saw us, he asked if we had seen anything. Eggy, pointed at me and said, *"He did it,"* and started laughing as if this were a joke. I pushed him and said, *"Shuddup, Eggy, I didn't do nuthin'."*

"Boys, stop playing," the cop said angrily, *"the girl is dead!"*

Dead! I didn't know she was dead! I thought she was just shot.

I looked at the cop. I could see tears running down his brown face. I never saw a cop cry before. *"We didn't see nuthin', sir."*

"Ok, boys," and he turned away, wiping his eyes.

Who could do this to Linda?

Albie went over to Linda's family. He came back and told us it was a guy robbing the store. Linda tried to stop him, and he shot her, just twenty minutes ago.

We waited for the ambulance to pick Linda up. The crowd grew larger. More cop cars showed up. My mother came *down with Cliff in the stroller, crying, "Oh God in heaven, Rick, that beautiful girl, she only did good, God bless her."*

When the ambulance came, we watched the drivers come out with a stretcher and place it on the floor next to Linda. They rolled her onto it. She seemed so limp, like a doll. I didn't understand why she didn't move or wake up. I saw red stains on her shirt, like ketchup, and her face was white like powder. Her eyes were closed. Her skin was smooth. She was so pretty, like an angel. How could she be dead? The ambulance drivers pulled a white sheet over her. They picked her up on the stretcher. Ramon, Linda's brother, helped to lift her.

I could hear Linda's mother weeping. I saw her with her family next to the stretcher. Some were holding and comforting her. When she saw the drivers carrying Linda to the back of the ambulance, she let out a wail and tried to go to her. Her family members restrained her, but she struggled free. She ran to Linda, pulling the white sheet off her, and wrapping her arms around her, picking her up and holding her, not ready to let her go.

"Linda, Linda!" she screamed. "Mi niña" (my child), "mi niña!" she howled, as if mortally wounded herself, kissing her, her tears running over the face of her daughter as she embraced her. She stroked her hair, and whispered to her, holding and pleading with her, as if she were still alive, still her little girl, asking her what had happened, as if she had only hurt herself, as if she could still bring her back. "Mi niña!" she screamed from such pain that I could hardly stand it. Many in the crowd, even people that never met her, began to cry. Some began praying out loud, saying Jesus' name. Some made the sign of the cross, what Linda tried to teach me once, and Mom almost brained me. Ramon slowly pulled his mother away. She clung to her little girl, not wanting to let her go. One of the drivers covered Linda's face again. The doors of the ambulance opened and swallowed up poor Linda, and they drove away.

My mother held me, as if to protect me, as if she were afraid that something like this could happen to my brothers or me, as if she were afraid to leave me alone in this place, the Bronx. She cried and said, "Oh, God in heaven, Ricky, how could this happen? How could this happen to our Linda? Who could do such a thing to that beautiful girl? It's terrible, such a tragedy, God help us!" She said, almost shouting. She looked at me and I could see the tears streaming down her face. "She was such a sweet girl, wasn't she, Ricky?"

"Yeah, Ma, she was."

She took my hand. "Come on, son." She pushed the stroller with Cliff in it, and we walked back home.

It was the second person I had seen killed in a few months.

Linda's family wore black for a week. My mother dropped off flowers to the family, but afterwards, we did not go back to Linda's house.

I always thought about Linda, how she smiled, her dimples, and how she helped me that time I cut my hand. I missed going to her house with all the people and loud music and funny smells from the kitchen. I didn't understand too much about death except that it meant I would never see her again. I didn't know where you went when you died, or if you could still talk or do things.

I wondered if she was with Jesus or if this would have even happened if she just believed in regular God, like the Jews did. A few days later, we were playing slug against the building and dodging cold water from the old people on the first floor.

-14-

My brother, Larry, called, the oldest of the brothers. "Hey, Rick, what's going on?" Larry was usually sunny in disposition, the good life of Florida resonant in his voice. But not today.

"What's the matter?" I asked.

"How's Mom doing?"

"She's OK, she opened her eyes today," I said seriously, as if a point of significance. "She's been sleeping non-stop, so she finally opened her eyes." I heard no response and continued: "When the kids visited, she opened her eyes and smiled. She hadn't opened her eyes in days."

"So she's not doing well?"

I thought I was delivering good news. ". . . Well, it's slow. Stroke is a different thing. It takes time."

"But she's OK? She's not in any danger?"

"No, she's not OK. She's had a serious stroke. She's bedridden. But I don't think she's in danger of dying."

"Oh," he said and then silence.

Larry was the quasi-father of our fatherless family, the leader of our motley band when we were young. He looked like Dad, combed his hair like Dad, and seemed big to us back then. He bought a car, went to college, got married, had kids, ran a factory, made money, all when we were very young. It was natural for us to look up to him. When we grew up, his Olympian stature may have diminished slightly, but the youthful impressions lingered, and Larry would always be first among us, the oldest.

"So how's Florida?" I asked, changing the topic.

"Great, Florida's great. Always warm. It's beautiful." Larry usually spoke this way, in short, truncated sentences, except when he was telling a joke where he displayed his verbal talents. He was also tough, amazingly tough.

"How's business?"

"So-so. It's OK." Did he sound morose because business was bad or because of Mom?

"How are Harold and Steven doing?" His kids were now fully grown, but always important as the first issue of our generation.

"They're good. Steven's getting married. Nice girl. Jewish. He's moving to Orlando."

"How's Harold?"

"He's living with us again." We were all very involved with Larry's kids, babysat them when they were infants, taught them things, playing the proud uncles. They were good kids, very respectful, still addressed us as Uncle so and so, almost an anachronism in this very informal age.

"How's Helen?" Of all Larry's achievements, marrying Helen was his greatest. This was a woman to build a life around: wonderful, nurturing, and highly intelligent. She wrote poetry, read, and was completely devoted to Larry, a throwback, almost, to another era of Jewish women. Her parents were Polish Jews and Holocaust survivors.

"She's good," said Larry, of the truncated sentence.

"Yeah?" I said as if to make sure. Helen was fragile, although I never realized how fragile early on, having idealized her as the perfect woman. She was the one who always cared for me as a child, fed me, or took me in when I cut school and hid out at their apartment on Pelham Parkway by Columbus High School where I went. She disapproved but did not challenge it; we talked for hours, she a receptive audience for my youthful, often radical ideas. Years later, she had become severely depressed, which shocked me; she the flawless flower of impeccable comportment, suddenly reeling. Her father, who had been institutionalized, died tragically in a fire, and this had shaken her frail soul. She had had issues with Mom, too, as all the daughters-in-law had.

"Yeah, she's good," Larry said.

Larry used to own a factory in the garment district in Manhattan, and he ran it like an autocrat. His employees lived in fear of him - but not just them, everyone. Sales people, vendors, retailers, everyone. He swore without remorse and did not suffer fools lightly. "You damn idiot" was a typical retort one might occasion to hear several times in the course of the day.

"You coming out with the boys?" I asked.

"No, I'll be out later."

"You sure?"

"Yeah," he said, with a trace of irritation. "How are your kids doing?" he asked, changing the topic.

"Good."

"So how'd this thing happen?"

I recited the invocation once more. ". . . Cholesterol, diabetes, and she was seventy eight."

"Awful, just awful," Larry said. I realized I was annoyed that he was not visiting.

I returned to the ICU and sat down at the nurse's station to look at my mother's chart. I reviewed the physician's orders. Dr. Regan had her on a heparin drip, Zocor (a cholesterol drug), pepcid (for acid reflux), and tenormin (for blood pressure). She received intravenous fluid at a rate of 100 cc/hour, and, except for ice chips, was NPO (nothing by mouth). This, of course, was gratuitous since she was unconscious.

There were no medicines unfortunately to dissolve the stroke or rejuvenate the damaged tissue. No charms to undo the harm. Short of such magic, we were left, instead, with the age-old methods of rehabilitation: the monotonous repetitions of flexing, extending, and re-educating errant muscles no longer willing to comply.

I skimmed through the pages of her chart, the endless scribbling of the well intentioned who could do nothing to help her, the wearisome medical record that was slowly gathering a weight of its own. Did the size of a chart, at some point, presage an utterly dismal outcome? Was there an equation that showed an inverse relationship between the size of a chart and the health of the patient?

There were other patients in the ICU, in various stages of debilitation: some chronic, some acute, some on life support – on a ventilator, comatose, invaded by all manner of lines, tubes, and catheters. The monitors hung over their beds in every room, little charged sentinels closely guarding their comings and goings; no irregularity, no blip in blood pressure, no change in heart rate, would go unnoticed. The nurses, too, watched carefully, tending to the wounded, adjusting IVs, and following the lines on the screens at the nurse's station.

What were her prospects? With the return of rudimentary movement came the small chance of restoring some semblance of normal life. I did not expect that she could ever live independently or carry on in the manner she was accustomed to – and this acknowledgement all but sickened me – but if she could relearn some basic movements, to stand and pivot, as in using a commode, or lifting a fork to her mouth, she could return home to live. I reconsidered the goals: stand and pivot, lifting a fork. I felt the familiar nausea returning as I contemplated my mother's post-stroke life.

I looked at my beeper, making sure it was on, a reflex after fifteen years of answering to this, my master.

What was it I hated more? Stroke or myself? Oddly, the question provoked a sense of appeasement. I had not answered it, but in thinking it, I seemed to feel better, my revulsion shifting to something more palatable. It was preferable to hate the disease.

A nurse walked by. "Can I help you, Dr. Moss?" She was young and attractive, dark blonde, of medium height, and a large diamond on a gold band circling her ring finger. She smiled at me, showing proper sympathy. I scanned the latest page of orders on my mother's chart. A white sheet covered by an assortment of scribbles pouring over the page and onto the next, courtesy of Dr. Regan.

"Is her PTT OK?" I asked. (PTT is a clotting test).

"I think it was a little lower than he wanted, so he increased the heparin."

"How is her blood pressure?"

"Running a little high."

"So he increased the tenormin?"

"Yes."

I leafed through the chart. It was growing ominously, like a tumor. Progress notes, consultations, flow sheets, orders, X-rays, labs, physical therapy: the full gamut of allied medical services brought to bear against her disease. The story was not uplifting; rather it was overwhelming: a dismal chronicle of an elderly woman sleeping continuously in a darkened, windowless, sanitized room. At what point did the numbing accumulation of data become superfluous? By some lights, Mom's chart was anemic. Still, it increased in size, day by day. I feared this tome: its weight, its dimension, its bulk. How then to stand athwart the offensive proliferation and shout, "Halt!" There was a simple answer: get her out of here and into my home.

I folded the chart and walked into her room, where she continued the day's chapter of the ongoing saga, the plot thus far unchanged. Her face was peaceful, as it had been. Her lip seemed to droop. I placed my hand over hers and observed her breathing. It was slow but rhythmic, the subtle movement of the chest discernible through the blanket. Her color was good, even pink, as it had always been before the stroke: alive and passionate, her robust face primed to match her vigorous personality. She hid nothing, was wired to her emotions directly, bypassing critical cortical influences that may have lead to more reasoned responses through the years.

I called out her name. Her eyelids fluttered. A flicker of recognition, and then, the faintest utterance: "Hi, Ricchh," as delivered by her unruly tongue. Incredible, I thought, she recognized me! Her first words since the sorry event now eight days ago. Could this be a forerunner of things to come? I smiled quickly enough for her glazed eyes to catch a glimpse before receding.

The blonde nurse walked in. "She's opening her eyes some, Dr. Moss," she said cheerfully.

"Well, yes, she just recognized me," I said exuberantly.

"She seems to be waking up a little," she said. She seemed decidedly less excited than I was.

"She just said my name."

"Uh huh."

"It's the first time since the stroke."

"She does speak Dr. Moss, just very little," she said casually.

"You mean she's spoken before?"

"Yes, very briefly and then she falls asleep."

"But she recognized me!" I said.

"Th-that's good, Dr. Moss," she said hesitantly.

"It is a positive sign."

"Y-yes, it's a positive sign."

"Is she moving?" I asked.

"Some."

"Really? Like what?"

"She squeezes my hand."

"Right and left?"

"No, only right."

She walked around to the head of the bed to adjust Mom's pillow. She checked her blood pressure and listened to her lungs. She took notes, to be transcribed later in Mom's ever-burgeoning chart. She seemed nervous with me in the room, perhaps conscious of the absurdity of her routines. After completing her visit, she looked at me and repeated the same phrase I had heard ad nauseam since the wretchedness began: "Vital signs are stable."

That was it. No uptick in emotion.

I watched her as she walked out. The mortuary-like atmosphere returned; my mother and I enfolded within it. She slept peacefully. Such an oddity. I confronted again these dreary moments at my mother's bedside, waiting patiently for some variation in the developing narrative. But the aseptic repetitions continued, her brief recognition of me, I now realized, a meaningless footnote. I sat numbly, holding her pulse, deriving some pleasure from its steady throbbing.

I contemplated the possibility of a nursing home, which, I realized, may be the epilogue to this. In general, I was not keen on them, particularly for Mom. They were, though, sometimes necessary and unavoidable - the thought of which I could barely stomach.

I looked at her and felt like saying something, like *how ya doing?* I gazed at the monitor, dumbly displaying numbers that showed her ship was still forging ahead. *Control bowel, stand and pivot, lift a fork.* A mantra.

I placed my hand on hers and thought of a distant but remarkably clear vision of an earlier chapter of her life – and its end. I closed my eyes and reminisced through the years . . .

My father hadn't visited us in the Bronx since he wrecked the kitchen. The brothers missed him, although we didn't miss the fighting. Without him there was peace in the house; at least, there were no major quarrels. There was no cursing, screaming, slapping, shoving, pushing, or throwing. There was normal family squabbling, predictable and pedestrian, but no violence.

When the doorbell rang that morning, a long ring, followed by the cigarette cough, we all knew who it was. Cliff and I ran to the door, followed by Jerry, the three youngest, still innocent enough to be excited when their Dad came home. Jack and Larry, the older ones, did not get up, suspicious of the sound, not yet ready to welcome their father back into the house. They stayed in their room, the one they shared, right next to the door. They remained sprawled on their beds. Mom was in the kitchen, making fijones (a Sephardic bean dish). She looked out from the kitchen when the door rang and recognized the cough. She didn't respond.

I unlocked the door and opened it. I saw, for the first time in months, my father, big and swarthy, a lit cigarette dangling from his lips. His jet-black hair was combed back; his left lip drooped as it always had from a prior bout with Bell's palsy. He wore a casual grey suit and black leather shoes. He pulled on his cigarette and blew out a stream of smoke. Then he grinned and said in his thick, cigarette voice, "How ya doin', monkeys?" And he opened his arms, laughing that low emphysematous laugh, picking Cliff and me up, roaring and blustery, like he had never left us. He put us down and bear-hugged Jerry. When Jack and Larry appeared hesitantly at the door, he swept them into his big arms, too.

"How my boys doin'?" he yelled. And he roared and hooted some more, poking and shoving his kids playfully. Cliff, in his three-year-old voice, asked, "Where ya been, Daddy?" And with this little comment, he picked Cliff up, smothering him with kisses, saying, "My little monkey, I missed you." Then he put him down, patted me on my head, put his hand on Jerry's shoulder, and pushed Jack and Larry, mock chal-

*lenging them, saying, "Ya dink ya ready for ya old man?"
They bobbed like boxers, trying to act tough. "C'mon," he
said, and guffawed some more, corralling his kids in a hearty
embrace. "I missed ya, boys," he said, and he continued jabbing and laughing with his little brood.*

*Then, after a pause, Dad looked around and asked for
Mom. "Where's yer mudda?" he said, staring at the cluster
of faces surrounding him. Mom had not bothered to come to
the door. We looked at each other uneasily.*

*"In the kitchen." We stood away, as Dad rushed past us
into the apartment, down the hallway, by the little bathroom
on the right, Jack and Larry's bedroom on the left, and into
the living room with the torn green couch that Mom slept
on. He passed the bedroom to the left where Cliff, Jerry, and
I slept, and walked to the kitchen, where Mom was stirring
a pot of fijones over a low flame. Dad stood at the entrance
to the kitchen. Mom did not lift her eyes, a blank expression
on her face.*

"Whatcha makin'?" Dad asked. Mom didn't answer.

*Dad looked at Mom and smiled. "How ya doin', kid?" he
asked pleasantly.*

Nothing.

*"I miss ya food, y'know." She stirred, looking up at him
briefly.*

"Ya look beautiful, Tilly."

And Mom smiled ever so faintly.

Dad stepped into the kitchen.

*Mom turned icy. "Don't step into this kitchen!" she
shouted suddenly. "How dare you come back here after nearly destroying it!"*

Dad backed out. "I-I'm sorry."

*"We don't need you around here anymore, you un-
derstand? Just send us money! Where's the money for last
week?"*

"I-I'm a little late, doll. I'm sor-"

"And the week before?"

"I know, Tilly, I'm behind, I'm sor-"

"*Whaddaya doin' with your money? Spending it at the track? At the bar? On your clothing?*" *she sneered disgustedly.* "*The kids gotta eat, y'know.*"

She returned to her pot, stirring it.

Dad leaned against the doorway. "*I got tickets for the circus,*" *he said.*

Mom kept stirring.

"*At da Garden.*"

"*The Garden?*" *she asked.*

"*Yeah, Madison Square Garden.*" *The brothers looked at each other incredulously.*

"*Ringling Brothers Barnum and Bailey!*" *he announced.*

The sneer on my mother's face lessened just slightly. She stopped stirring the pot and said, "*Really?*"

"*Yeah, doll.*"

"*For everyone?*" *Mom asked.*

"*Everyone.*"

"*How are we getting there?*" *Her mood was lighter.*

"*In my DeSoto.*"

"*Ya mean we're driving?*"

Dad smiled. "*Yeah, I got a new car.*"

Mom did not ask him how he paid for the car, or how he could buy a car and not send money for the kids, or how much money he gambled or drank away or spent frivolously on clothing. She did not ask where he spent his time and why he hadn't visited in several months. She preferred instead to suspend judgment and be swept along by the excitement of the moment, perhaps hoping against hope for a reprieve, a new chance at happiness.

"*You really have tickets, Harry,*" *she asked, saying his name for the first time.*

And Dad, sensing victory, looked at her and smiled his crooked smile, his swagger returning. "*Yeah, doll, don't worry 'bout a 'ding.*"

With this, Dad turned to face his sons. "*Ya ready to have fun, kids?*" *he asked triumphantly.*

"*Yeah,*" *we shouted back ecstatically.*

Mom turned off the flame and covered the pot. She took her apron off and walked out of the kitchen, past the living room and to the hallway closet where she kept her clothes. She pulled out stockings, a dress, and shoes. She went to the bathroom and reappeared transformed: face made up, eyelashes, lipstick, pretty dress, hat, high heels, and glowing. We hurried down the stairs, looking for Dad's Desoto, the big black car with the chrome and tail fins.

"Oh, Harry," Mom said, as if in a trance, and we piled into the car.

Mom sat next to Dad in the front, along with Cliff by the window. The other four of us squeezed into the back. We opened the windows, locked the doors, and Dad started the car. He moved into the street, winding his way to the highway. He turned on the radio, and we drove downtown.

Manhattan was an exotic place for us, like visiting another planet. The tall buildings, the narrow streets, the massive throngs, and snarling traffic were exhilarating. Dad parked the car and we traversed the avenues, skipping, racing, jumping, and finally coming upon the great arena, Madison Square Garden.

We stood in line, passed through the gate and entered another world. It was grand, the crowd teeming and thunderous, the atmosphere electric. There were clowns, fire breathers, sword swallowers, lion tamers, elephants, horses, camels, bears, trapeze artists, acrobats, snake charmers, and contortionists, a splashy, rousing, three-ring circus in New York City. Then it was over, and we went home. We piled back into the car and drove back to the Bronx.

Dad was still smiling when he pulled out his cigarettes, Camel cigarettes, unfiltered. He lit one up. He was proud of his Camels, bragged about them, told us they were the best cigarettes in the world. He inhaled deeply, enjoying the flavor, then exhaled, letting out a stream of smoke. He flicked the cigarette into the ashtray, and then left it there, the lit edge depositing an ash, the red circle advancing, smoke wafting up, curving, folding, gathering above our heads, forming a dense cloud. He picked up the cigarette again, dragged on it, and put it down. As the car filled with cigarette smoke, my mother began to frown. She blinked once or twice. The brothers were quiet in the back, looking out at the traffic, the buildings, and the ships in the Hudson River. Dad dragged on his cigarette. Then he extinguished it. He looked around. "Ya kids have a good time?"

"Yeah, Dad."

"I didn' hear no one say 'danks,'" *he said.*

"Thanks, Dad."

He laughed. "Ya sound tired. Yul be ready fa sleep whenya get home."

And we continued the drive.

He reached into his shirt pocket for another smoke. He jerked the pack up, delivering a cigarette through the opening, grabbing it with his lips. My mother frowned again. Halfway through the cigarette, Cliff, sitting next to Mom, coughed. Mom looked at Dad. Cliff coughed again. Mom turned. "Your smoke is bothering him, Harry."

"Ok, I'll open da window." *He opened it a crack, and the cool air entered the car and felt good. He continued pulling on his cigarette. Cliff coughed again. And he wiped his eyes.*

"Could you stop smoking, Harry? I think it's bothering him."

Dad looked at Mom, taking another drag. "Naw, he's OK. Here, just open da window." *And he leaned across Mom and Cliff's lap and opened Cliff's window.*

He kept smoking. Smiling. When he finished this cigarette, he pulled out another. He hawked up a thick gob, opened the window, and spit it out. "You kids like da circus?"

"Yeah, Dad."

And we continued the drive up to the Bronx.

Dad was blowing smoke rings in the car. "Hey, kids, ya see dat?"

Mom frowned and said, "Harry, I can't take the smoke. Could you please stop smoking?" *She looked at Dad.* "Smoking isn't good for you, ya know," *she said.*

Dad half smiled. He tossed the cigarette out the window.
And Mom was content. Dad opened the window a little more
and the smoke seemed to clear.

A few minutes later, Mom asked Dad what his plans were.
"Whaddaya mean, doll?" Dad answered good-naturedly.

"I mean what are you going to do?"

"About what?"

"A-About the family?"

"Ya mean da money?"

"Yes. But not just the money. I mean the family."

Dad didn't say anything at first "Uhh, let's see, doll,"
he said finally.

Mom frowned.

A few minutes passed. Mom said, "Rick needs orthope-
dic shoes."

"Huh?"

"Orthopedic shoes."

"What's he need dat for?"

"He's flat-footed."

"He runs like a horse, dis kid, whaddaya mean flat-foot-
ed?"

"He has no arch. And he's pigeon toed. His ankles fold
in."

"Whodahelltolyadat?"

"The foot doctor."

"Whut is he, some kind a nut? Dis kid runs like a horse,
I tolya, he climbs trees like a monkey. Whooya takin' my kids
ta."

"A foot specialist at Bronx Lebanon."

"Dis kid wuz ridin' a bike when he wuz four. He's an
animal. Dere ain't nothin' wrong wit his feet."

"They cost 48 dollars."

Dad's eyes widened. "Yoo outta your mind?"

A few minutes later, Dad was smoking again. Hacking,
puffing. No one peeped. Then Cliff said, "Mommy, I don't
like Daddy smoking."

    Mom looked at Dad. "I asked you nicely to stop smoking."

    Dad said, "Jus' open the window, Tilly." Mom opened the window again, but Cliff continued to cough.

    "You just have to stop smoking, Harry."

    "Doll, we're almost there."

    "You're inconsiderate."

    "Awright, awready." He opened the window and threw the cigarette out.

    "You know I don't like it when you smoke."

    He said nothing.

    "Why do I have to beg you like a child? You're worse than the kids."

    Dad shook his head. Mom stared. Dad ignored her.

    "If you stopped smoking maybe you'd have money for the kids."

    Dad said nothing.

    "And this car. Where'd you get the money for this?"

    Dad shook his head.

    "And the circus. You've got money for a circus, but nothing for your kids!"

    Dad took a deep smokeless breath. "Doll, we had a good time, didn' we?"

    "That's not the point."

    "Whut point? Cancha jus' relax?"

    "With no money and five kids?"

    "Awright, awready."

    "You smoke. You drink. You gamble. You spend your money on cars you can't afford – and you don't have sixty lousy dollars a week for your kids!"

    He coughed and lit up another cigarette. Mom grabbed the pack of cigarettes, crumbled them up, and threw them out the window. Cliff started crying. Mom grabbed the cigarette dangling from his mouth and threw it out the window. "Selfish sonofabitch!" she said. Dad didn't say anything. "You're selfish. Do you understand? Selfish!" Mom shouted.

    "Shuddup awready, nag, nag, nag!" Dad yelled back.

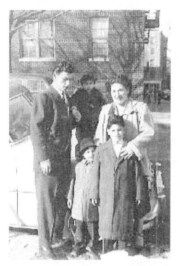

"Don't talk to me that way!" She jabbed her index finger at him, almost poking him. "Where do you get off talking that way in front of your kids?" Dad shook his head, pressing his lips, and then slowed to pull off the highway. The shouting stopped, and the car plunged into silence. The city streets were dark.

We got off on the Arthur Avenue exit, drove up 175th street, turned on to Crotona Park North, and approached the front of our building. I looked at the little stone lions on either side of the staircase, the small courtyard, the number 867 written over the entrance. Dad stopped the car. There was silence. Dad stared out the front windshield. He reached absentmindedly for another cigarette, but remembered Mom had tossed them out.

"Come on, kids," Mom said, opening the door. "Be careful, Ricky," she said to me, making sure there were no cars coming. We trudged toward the house, not sure whether to thank Dad or even to say goodbye. I heard Mom slam the door. She followed quickly behind us. Dad turned to look at her, as if wanting to say something. I wished he would. I heard Mom whimpering as she hurried past. I looked at Dad. He turned away and shook his head. Then he drove off.

The nurse walked in, interrupting my reverie. "I have to turn your mother, Dr. Moss," she said. She looked at me and smiled. I held my mother's hand for a moment. I kissed her and left.

-15-

When I returned to my office, I reflected again on the consequences of this disease. It was a different sort of illness, really, an oddity in the world of disease, unique in its abruptness. It rendered its victims invalids immediately and without warning, transforming wholly functioning individuals into bedridden convalescents – and with no obvious cause, as if overtaken by evil spirits.

Consider its impact: an individual otherwise fully autonomous, engaged in all manner of activity, converted, quite suddenly, into a cripple unable to manage the most basic tasks. It was an abrupt rupture in the weave of one's life, a sudden and crude ousting from the boundaries of normal routine, and into a therapeutic netherworld of bedpans and diapers - all in the blinking of an eye. The cause remained hidden within the waves and filaments of the brain, buried deep within its substance: a ludicrous crumb lodged in a vessel, a crumb so small that it would hardly be noticed could it have been laid out somehow to see, a worthless fragment, yet capable of unleashing the bleakest of harvests.

No other disease process had such overwhelming effect. None had the power to confiscate so decisively one's capacity to act. It was the profoundest of dislocations, save for death itself.

And what was the result of such devastation on the individual? Compare, if you will, the impact of the other great scourges of modern life: cancer and heart disease. Even the dread diagnosis of malignancy, with its terrible psychological consequences, the fear and horror of it all, the unending tests, X-rays, biopsies, scans, and the violence of its treatments, its chemotherapy, radiation, and debilitating surgery. Yet, at least, cancer left its victims with faculties intact until its end stages. One could carry on, engaged in the usual routines, making end of life preparations, doing special things with loved ones, all quite feasible until the final weeks or months.

Heart attacks, too, assuming one survived the initial assault, left the individual still able to manage, albeit more cautiously; or any other chronic debilitating illness that wound irrevocably towards death. One still had time to act and function, to direct affairs, before the disease's grip curled too tightly in its final surges. But a stroke was different. It struck at the core – the brain - and left it reeling and unable to minister. It cleaved and shattered without warning.

There was a note by my phone. "Call the librarian," it said. Good. I dialed her extension. She had some articles for me. But the women had already picked them up she said. Ah, they forgot to remove the note. I looked over by the mail and found several of them. One immediately caught my eye. On "Vinpocetine." Such a name. More like an Italian actor or opera singer, especially if the final 'e' were changed to an 'i'. It was, in fact, a "neuroprotective" agent. The article was from Europe, with contributors from Sweden, Hungary, and Italy, a multinational force. I skimmed through it. It ended, as many medical articles seemed to, with the exhortatory call for *"further studies to understand the mechanism of action and to determine its therapeutic efficacy in the clinical setting."*

Vinpocetine had been used effectively for organic brain syndrome since 1978, making it a real old timer, consistent, I supposed, with the condition it treated. Of late, researchers experimented for possible use in the stroke patient. It was "neuroprotective" in that it blocked sodium channels. But that was not the focus of the article. It was found also to increase cerebral circulation, and, specifically, to improve blood flow to the "peri-stroke" area. This meant that nerve cells teetering on irreversible damage in and around the infarct itself might be saved. It offered the promise of improved outcomes – based on further study. This, the endless refrain, and therefore, of no immediate use. I tossed it on the pile covering my desk.

The laws of nature were stacked heavily against the stroke patient, and yet, there they were, diligent minds attempting to manipulate the physiologic variables to squeeze out a shard of hope where none existed: a dismal sort of alchemy, I thought, as likely as transforming lead into gold. The laws of nature were unforgiving, and the chances for success poor. If it were otherwise, strokes would be reversed by a wish and a pinch of pixie dust. In the meantime, I would hover pathetically over their efforts, a ghoulish bystander entwined in their struggle by my own fictions, hoping for some morsel despite the odds.

There was another article, something about Clomethiazole. I put it in my bag to look at later. For now, my mother and I were left with the old remedies. Yet, I derived some pleasure in learning about the efforts of the gallant who battled this disease - I, now a loyal partisan of the anti-stroke faction, engaged, at least vicariously, in the long campaign of attrition against an implacable foe. I shut the lights in my office and left. It was not all futile, I told myself.

It was a few minutes before five and I wanted to catch the radiologist before he left. I rushed over to the

X-ray department and asked the clerk to pull my mother's MRI scan. The clerk was an attractive blonde with glazed eyes, almost dizzy, I thought, and a breathy voice. She seemed totally out of place in this midwestern community hospital, working as a clerk in a purple uniform, pulling films for grizzled doctors. She should have been a model somewhere or an actress. "Here you are, Dr. Moss," she said.

I walked into the office of Dr. Fred Mehringer, a radiologist on staff. "I was sorry to hear about your mother, Rick," he said, pulling the films from the folder. Fred had been at the hospital for more than twenty-five years, one of the good ole boys. He had a mustache, light beard, graying hair, and was overweight. "Your mother had no history of vascular disease, did she?"

"None," I answered.

"Too bad," he added sympathetically, as he began studying the films, slice-by-slice, surveying the cross sections of my mother's brain that appeared before us as images of black, gray, and white. Amidst the undulations of brain matter, a whitish flare appeared in one of the images, in the medial horn of her right temporal lobe.

"That's where it begins, Rick," said Fred, pointing his chubby finger. We continued, watching the white flare grow larger, becoming more prominent, reaching deeper into brain tissue, becoming, finally, a tear shaped opacity about the size of an almond.

"That's it, Rick, at it's biggest."

And big it was, considering the real estate.

"What structures are we talking about?" I asked.

"Basal ganglia, mainly."

"What do they do?"

"They're the deep nuclei, relay centers, deal with emotions," he said.

I could tell nothing about that, as she had been asleep since the stroke. "What else did it affect?"

"The internal capsule. Those are the nerve fibers that control muscle activity and movement."

"That's what caused the paralysis."

"Yep."

"Anything else?" I asked.

"Some mild cortical atrophy, micro-ischemic disease, pretty typical for her age."

I looked at the white tear-shaped shadow that fell across the inner half of my mother's right cerebral hemisphere and felt as if I were at the scene of a crime.

"Any hemorrhage?"

"No, there's no distortion or midline shift, it's an ischemic infarct," he said.

It seemed harmless enough. Yet this white shadow on a strip of film had exposed a disaster.

"Any swelling?"

"No, not really."

"No mass effect – swelling or compression?" I asked.

"No."

The white shadow. This was the area of "infarct." I wondered what thoughts had originated there, in the realm of the white shadow. What impulses had shuttled along that dense circuitry en route to the spinal cord and yonder, to muscle fibers afield, that allowed her to speak, and walk, or hold my hand?

Within the target area, the killing field, the *ground zero* of this catastrophe, there had once been the yammer of electro-chemical discourse, the eternal nerve chatter that allowed for the miracle of movement. And those sparks had flashed and spun through that maze of now rotted nerve fiber that showed up as white on celluloid. It was a crime, a terrible crime, and we were here now, Fred and I, at the scene of the crime, looking over the corpses of dead nerve cells, whited out and congealed, their bodies stiff and decaying, wondering how it had happened, who had done it, and what the motive was.

"So what causes this, Fred?" I asked.

"*You* know, Rick, the usual culprits, cholesterol, blood pressure, vascular disease."

"She was always so healthy."

"A shame. How old is she?"

"Seventy eight."

"It happens, Rick."

"You've seen them this big?"

"Oh, yeah, I've seen 'em."

He nodded and tightened his lips to emphasize the point, rubbing his soft underbelly.

I pondered the unhappy micro event once more. It had occurred in the deep hollows of my mother's brain; the development of plaque in the wall of a vessel, the rupture of that plaque, the cascade of reactions that lead to the formation of a thrombus that shut down circulation, starving the cells, strangling them, throwing them into a death heave, gripped by hypoxia, unable to digest sugars, unable to create energy to drive the cellular machinery, the cells drowning in the waste products of their own metabolism. It was a tragic and brutal death of nerve cell and supporting tissue at the hands of a tiny criminal, an atherosclerotic plaque, aided and abetted by a cast of unseemly characters – platelets, fibrin, red blood cells, and others.

"Would you call it a major stroke," I asked Frank despondently.

"Yes, Rick, I'm afraid so."

"It's not massive though?"

"No, not massive, but major."

"You've seen them bigger?"

"I've seen *whiteouts,* Rick, half the brain gone with no warning, carotid thrombosis, just like that." He snapped his fingers and snorted, the little hairs in his nostrils flipping in and out of his nose. "She should recover her speech," he added.

But control bowel, stand and pivot, lift a fork?

He looked at the films, a satisfied expression on his hairy face. He was happy in his little world of celluloid and shadow, far removed from the gritty unfathomables of flesh and blood, of heart attacks, strokes, and tumors. It was a well-manicured lawn of a world.

"Thanks, Fred," I said.

"Sorry, Rick."

When I arrived home, I played with my kids, had dinner, read them a story, and put them to bed. I did not rush through my paternal responsibilities, nor did I dally. I performed them as diligently as established routine required. But when completed, I immediately descended to my study like a thief. I was eager to pick up the last article I had brought home from the office. I did not expect much from it, but my need to know more was great. Would there be some new therapy to get my mother to sit up, put her clothes on, and walk out of the hospital? I sat back in my swivel chair and began to read.

This one was from the American Heart Association on Clomethiazole, another neuroprotective agent, with all the inherent limitations. From what I had read elsewhere, this, too, would be of no benefit, the sacred "time window" and all that. As it turned out, even when used within the limited time constraints, Clomethiazole was a dismal failure, the article almost proclaiming it. *"Clomethiazole does not improve outcome in patients with ischemic stroke,"* it announced glumly. The paper began with the obligatory dirge about stroke being the third leading cause of death and the leading cause of disability in the country with 700,000 new strokes occurring each year. It was a randomized, double blind, multicenter, placebo-controlled study involving nearly 1200 patients. It failed to show any benefit for its molecular champion (Clomethiazole). I applauded their honesty.

There was a final editorial comment by an Australian professor who wondered if the drug would be more effective if married to TPA. He thought that TPA could serve as a vehicle to deliver the drug ever deeper into the more ominous regions of the infarct, into the ischemic penumbra: that frangible border of dying tissue surrounding the necrotic center. It was here where many researchers hung their hopes. Perhaps, the writer postulated, ushered in on the wing of the intrepid TPA, Clomethiazole, its neuroprotective bride, could be delivered more effectively to the dying cells. He wrote this, it seemed, to allay the disappointment of the researchers at their failure to discover "The Next Great Drug," something of the order of, "no worries, mates, some good will come of it." It was all very collegial, but for now, they had succeeded only in discovering what not to do, a kind of negative progress.

I tossed the paper on a shelf and observed the spinning of the fan above me. My efforts for the day were done. I was not despondent, but apathy instead had found me. My mother remained as she was, and so did I, neither of us closer to our objectives than before. I lived now in a state of chronic abnormalcy, and realized that this, too, was becoming routine, the adaptive mechanisms already at work. In time, I would come to see all this as normal, and the thought alarmed me.

I went outside to the patio near the small pond with Japanese fish swimming amidst the brown and copper colored rocks, the sounds of the little waterfall, and the crickets nearby in the forest. Ying was there, tending her flowers. I said nothing to her and sat down, a glass of iced tea in my hand. We always enjoyed these final minutes of the day, amidst the flowers and sounds, a reprieve, an oasis of peace before sleep.

I visited Mom with Noah and Arielle the next morning in her telemetry bed. The nurse was in the room with Mom, doing "neuro checks." When we walked in, Mom turned slightly, and smiled. This, to me, bordered on an epiphany (and I did not care if the nurses were cavalier). She then returned her attention to the nurse, as if it were all in a day's work. I kept the children quiet and allowed the nurse to complete her routine.

"Eyes are open, speech is slurred," she said.

I listened.

"She is more alert today, Dr. Moss."

"Good," I said.

"Grab my fingers, Mrs. Moss," the nurse said, placing her fingers in Mom's right hand. "That's it," she said, as Mom grasped the nurse's fingers with her one functioning hand. The nurse then shifted to Mom's left hand and asked her to grip them. Nothing.

"Moderate to weak on the right, absent on the left. Still no movement on the left, Dr. Moss," she said, marking her flow sheet. She continued. "Arm and leg movement about the same, weak to moderate on the right, absent on the left."

I nodded obediently once more.

I glanced at Mom's chart. Her oxygen saturation was 96%, which was good. Her respirations were "unlabored and symmetric," and the EKG monitor showed normal sinus rhythm.

The nurse flashed a penlight into Mom's eyes. "Pupils equal and reactive," she said. I nodded again as she checked off another box on the flow sheet.

"Not much change, Dr. Moss, but a little more alert."

"Good," I nodded, controlling myself. She continued writing.

"Ok," the nurse said as she completed her notes, "she's all yours."

I moved to her bedside. "How are you, Mom," I said, feeling elated. I was pleased (delighted!) she was awake.

She nodded and said, "O-chhay." Slurred, but, at least, something.

"You were sleeping for days, you know."

She nodded weakly.

"Ok, kids, come over and say hello." Arielle and Noah hesitantly approached. Kids were funny about old people; they did not like to kiss them, or like the way they looked or smelled. We were the same growing up. I remembered Mom threatening us if we did not kiss her mother hello. "Hi, Nona," Noah said meekly. Then, Arielle, too, contributed a timorous smile and greeting.

Mom actually broke into a crooked smile, the left half missing, but a smile just the same. I was thrilled.

"You look better, Mom," I said.

"Yeah, Nona," said Arielle, finding her voice.

"You're not blowing bubbles any more," said Noah, remembering again Mom's garbled efforts to speak the evening she had the stroke. I laughed.

"That's good. Now tell Nona what you're doing today."

"I'm going to violin," Arielle said.

"Me, too," said Noah.

Mom raised her right eyebrow. She reached out with her right hand to hold Arielle.

"I made you a picture, Nona," Arielle said, "at synagogue." She unfolded a piece of paper. "It's for Rosh Hashanah," she said, the Jewish New Year coming in a couple of weeks. It was a crayon drawing of a Shofar (the ram's horn), a Jewish star, and some of the letters of the Hebrew alphabet on a background of sparkly green stuff.

"Gchood," Mom said. Arielle smiled.

Noah, though, was not thrilled. "What about me?" he said.

And Mom gave him the gift of a crooked smile as well.

"Do you need anything, Ma?" I asked.

She shook her head.

"You want something to drink?"

This time she nodded.

"Is it OK?" I wondered aloud. She was NPO (nothing by mouth). But what harm would a sip of water do?

I found a cup and straw and filled it with water. I held it to my mother's lips as she took a sip through the straw. Just a small sip. A moment later, she coughed. And coughed again. And she kept on coughing. A lot of coughing for a single sip. It *wasn't* OK. As if to accentuate that, the nurse walked in. "She's NPO, Dr. Moss," she said admonishingly. "Nothing by mouth except ice chips."

I nodded, feeling roguish and dumb.

"Dr. Regan ordered an NG feeding tube," she said. "Her barium swallow showed she's still aspirating."

I remembered Dr. Regan telling me about that. He asked me if I wanted a feeding gastrostomy tube placed. I told him no at the time.

"Can you get me some ice chips, then?" I asked.

"Sure."

So, Mom enjoyed a few ice chips that I dutifully spooned into her mouth (the children watching the grim spectacle solemnly), a simple pleasure for someone who had always relished her food.

We stayed a little longer, chatted, and then it was time to go. Mom was getting tired and the kids growing impatient. But it was a good visit, the best since it had all began.

"OK, Mom, we'll be in tomorrow."

The kids lined up and kissed her with only minimal nudging. "Goodbye, Nona," they said. Then something reminded me . . .

When I was a kid, I never thought much about fire-escapes, the metal platforms attached to the sides of buildings under our window with ladders zigzagging down to the ground floor. Some of the buildings had them in the front,

some in the back, but every building in the Bronx had them. People used the fire escape for many different things. Some hung their laundry. Some put little stoves there and had cookouts. Some listened to music. Some talked to others on their fire escapes from floor to floor or even building to building. Some threw firecrackers and cherry bombs off the fire escapes. Some dumped water on noisy kids in the street below. I saw a lot of things that people did on their fire escapes, but I never saw anyone escape from a fire.

Mom didn't mind us playing on the fire-escape. Sometimes she became nervous when we went down the fire escape to Dennis on the second floor or up the fire escape to see Robert and his brother, Frank, on the fourth floor. They just moved from West Virginia. Hicks from West Virginny, Mom called them. "Be careful, Ricky, watch your step," she yelled, when I climbed out the window. "If you get hurt, I'll brain ya."

"OK, Ma."

"And watch your little brother."

There was nothing special that happened on the fire escape, except for the time the guy with the greasy hair came by. I never saw this guy before. I never knew how he got there, if he climbed up from the ground or down from the roof. His eyes were red, and he kept wiping his nose on his sleeve. He had a Spanish accent, like Linda's brother, Ramon.

It was almost dark when Mom, Cliff, and I got home with the groceries. It was dark in the house because Mom had all the lights out; she also closed and locked the windows. Mom started locking the windows since the night of bloody murder and after Linda got shot. She closed the door behind her as we entered and locked it, two locks and a chain. She opened the light and asked if anyone was home. No one answered. We walked inside, and I helped Mom with the bags.

There was a noise from the kitchen. We could not see because it was dark, but we all heard it. It sounded like the window. I looked at Mom. I wanted to leave. I wanted to undo the locks and chain and leave. But Mom stood there listening.

Then we heard the noise again, like someone trying to pry open the window; then someone banging the window, and then someone yelling, "Sheet, mun!" I begged Mom to leave, but instead she walked down the hall towards the kitchen.

"Mom, let's get outta here," I cried. Then I heard the window break and glass crashing on the floor. I screamed and Cliff started crying. Mom didn't look at us or try to comfort us. She walked into the kitchen where the noise came and picked up an empty coke bottle from beside the refrigerator. Then she switched on the light. We looked up and saw a man with dark, greasy hair, standing outside on the fire escape. He was holding a flashlight. He glared at us through the broken window, a look of surprise on his face as if he was wondering what we were doing in our house.

Mom didn't say anything. What she did was she threw the bottle right through the window, splattering the glass all over the guy, his face and hair, and the kitchen floor below him.

"Ahhh, sheet, mun," he screamed angrily, wiping the flecks and chips from his face and spitting. He glared at us angrily. He was about to climb through the shattered window when Mom grabbed a kitchen knife from the sink. He stopped and looked at Mom holding the knife. "Are you crazee, ladee?" he said. His eyes were red and swollen, his nose was running, and he kept wiping it on his sleeve. He still had small particles of glass on his face and body. Mom gripped the knife and stared at him. Her eyes were two tiny black dots. "Crazee beetch," he said. Mom walked towards the broken window, the knife in her hand, while Cliff and I cowered behind her, crying hysterically.

"Are you crazee, ladee?" the guy said. Mom stared at the guy, her hand shaking and white around the knife, only a broken windowpane separating them. His face was ugly and pocked, and his lower lip twitched. He wiped his nose repeatedly. He reached for something in his back pocket. I screamed. He looked at me and at Mom. He sneered. He kicked the window, breaking some more glass. He cursed and spat. Then he

said, "Ah, sheet, mun." He turned and grabbed the rail of the fire escape and climbed down the metal stairs. We heard his footsteps and his voice, "Sheet, mun," we heard him say. He jumped to the first floor and down the ladder to the alley below. Then we heard the footsteps of someone running.

We stood there in the kitchen with the broken glass on the floor. I looked at Mom, and she looked at me. Cliff stopped crying. Mom was shaking but calm. Then, she said, "Damn neighborhood," and she swept the glass from the floor.

-16-

I stopped by the nurse's station at telemetry before seeing Mom this morning, nine days post stroke. I reviewed the chart. Dr. Regan had written that the MRI scan had shown an infarct of the internal capsule that would ". . . adversely affect her rehabilitation." He added under his assessment that she had a ". . . dense left hemi paralysis."

I noted that he had stopped the oxygen monitor and started her on an aspirin suppository (she was unable to swallow a pill). He had placed a foley catheter to empty her bladder, as she was incontinent and had ordered a "skilled care evaluation," which was preparatory for her being transferred to the skilled care unit. He had also written to move her to the third floor, which meant she would be leaving telemetry. There was also a note from the speech therapist, who said she would continue monitoring her "swallowing." For the time being, she had recommended Mom consume nothing more than ice chips.

I walked into her room to see her. She was lying in bed, eyes open and alert. She greeted me with her right eye, raising her right eyebrow. he lifted her right arm in a sort of wave.

"How are ya, Mom?"

She nodded as if to say, "OK."

"So, they're moving you out of telemetry."

The nurse in the room said, "We'll miss her, too." Mom smiled.

"So how's she doing?" I asked.

"She's stable, vital signs are good. Neurologically, she is about the same. Her left side is still flaccid," said the nurse.

"No movement?"

"None, I'm afraid."

I looked at the flow sheet. The nurse had recorded, "...sinus rhythm, breath sounds clear, left side flaccid, able to take ice chips only, incontinent large amount of urine, perianal care given, slurred but appropriate speech..." as pithy a summary as any, this, the day's entry for the chronicle of my mother's new life.

I sat with Mom and we talked, and I watched her, and she seemed OK. She was going to the regular floor today and was going to have an NG tube placed. Speech therapy was planning to follow her. Skilled care would evaluate her for what I assumed would be a long stay.

When I arrived in my office, I noticed an article on my desk, *"The Arithmetic of Stroke."* Clever, really, the title, suggesting, as it did, that the complex topic of stroke could be broken down into simple arithmetic. I began to read it. It was deceptively ponderous (considering the title), yet another moribund chapter in the mushrooming literature on stroke.

My nurse walked in, informing me that the first patient had arrived. I read quickly. The concept was simple enough: *disturbance in blood flow over duration.* Below a certain level of flow, irreversible damage occurred within minutes. Above that level, a return of function was still possible provided the duration was not too long. Instead of minutes, the time frame might be hours. The center of the stroke, the infarct, was beyond repair, but the *penumbra* of the stroke, the peristroke area, was where opportunity rested. If we could influence favorably one or both of these variables, then a return from the brink for ischemic but still viable tissue was possible. This conceptualization had a surprising effect on me. I became agitated.

I called my nurse. "Get Dr. Braun, please."

What agents were available that could take advantage of this, I wondered? I felt my pulse quicken.

"Dr. Braun is on line 1, Dr. Moss."

I picked up. "Jason, got a minute?"

"Yes, Rick, of course."

"What can you tell me about Vinpocetine?"

"Oh, it's been around, an old drug, used for organic brain syndrome."

"What about stroke?"

"I don't know about that."

"I read something out of Europe. It said that it increased circulation to the peristroke tissue."

He took a deep breath. "Well, perhaps, but it was probably experimental. In any event, it is not available in this country."

"It is good for up to five days past the stroke."

"Well, perhaps, but still not available."

"But the concept is valid. Reducing the total number of dead nerve cells," I said.

"Yes, of course, it is valid, *in theory*, but how to achieve that in practice is the question."

"There are so many drugs for improving circulation, but nothing for stroke?"

"Nothing proven. Only TPA."

"What about Clomethiazole?"

"A failure. A big study. Nothing came of it. It was no better than placebo, maybe worse."

"How about combining it with TPA?"

"It's been suggested, but not studied. I doubt it will make a difference. And, in any case, not useful in your mother's setting. She is beyond the time."

"So, what then?"

"Only therapy," he said.

"No agents? No stroke-busting drugs. I read something about osteogenic protein – out of Harvard."

"Yes, it encouraged neural sprouting – but only in animal studies."

"But it could be given at any time."

"True, there are no time constraints," he agreed.

"It dealt only with the surviving cells, promoted neural reorganization," I said.

"Yes, the concept is good."

"The whole idea is good. It gets away from time constraints."

"Correct . . ."

"and deals with whatever healthy cells are left – *after* the stroke."

"I know, but still experimental."

"Treatment window may be weeks instead of hours!"

"Yes."

"What about axonal growth factor to promote the branching of nerve fibers?" I asked.

"Still in the research phase – like osteogenic protein."

I looked at my quivering right hand throttling the neck of the phone. I happened to notice the painting of the Buddha on the wall, surrounded by the circle of flames with hands cupped and resting on folded ankles, his eyes turned inward.

"You know I am very frustrated."

"I know that, Rick."

My nurse appeared at the door to tell me we now had two patients.

"So there is nothing beyond the usual prescriptions?" I asked, more calmly.

"I'm afraid not."

"Alright, Jason, thanks."

I hurried to my patients . . .

When I went to see Mom in her new room on the medical ward, she already had the NG tube in place. "Hi, Mom," I said, as I entered the room. She was resting, but opened her eyes upon hearing my voice. She waved apathetically with her right hand and half smiled. "So they've got you all hooked up now," I said.

There was something disconcerting about seeing her with an NG tube running out of her nose. It came with a bag of white creamy liquid hanging from a pole next to her bed.

"Did it hurt when they passed the tube?" I asked.

"No." She shook her head.

"You feel any better now that you're getting some food?"

She shrugged. "It's occhay."

I read the chart. The barium swallow did not look good.

"*. . . was found to exhibit a moderate-severe dysphagia,*" read the note, "*recommend nothing by mouth with non-oral nutrition . . .*"

"At least they got you out of the ICU."

As if to punctuate the last remark, a nurse walked in. Middle aged, stout, and friendly. She had cared for many of my patients through the years.

"So this is your mother, Dr. Moss?" she said. "She's a very nice lady."

She adjusted her pillow. "Here, hon," she said, gently tucking it under Mom's head. She checked her blood pressure and heart rate. "Looks good." She placed a syringe in the NG tube and pulled back. "No residual. We can increase the feeding." She smiled as she dialed in a higher rate on the pump. "She seems to be tolerating the NG tube feedings well."

"No diarrhea?"

"No."

"Good." Again, I noted the absurd increments by which we measured progress in the universe of stroke.

"So your Mom was visiting when this happened?"

"Yes."

"That's too bad. She was telling me."

"So, she's speaking more."

"Yes, she is. In the morning especially." The nurse seemed bubbly. She stood next to Mom, fingering her necklace. A silver Jewish star and a jade amulet. One a gift from Jerry, the other from Ying. She was careful to place the Jewish star in front.

"It's beautiful, Mrs. Moss."

"Thancchs," she said, and smiled, proud of her Jewish star, her badge of honor.

"The barium swallow did not look good," I said.

"No, I saw that. She'll get better, though, Dr. Moss," sounding an optimistic note. "They'll start therapy tomorrow," she added.

"Did speech therapy come by?"

"Yes, there's a report in the chart."

I looked for it.

The same specialist that had done the barium swallow had written it. "*. . . found to exhibit severe dysarthria with receptive and expressive language deficits...*"

"About the same," I remarked.

"Yes. But the therapy will help."

"Have you seen much progress with strokes like this?"

"Yes, sometimes," she nodded affirmatively.

I continued reading: "*long term goals: Patient will utilize functional speech, language, swallowing abilities 90% of the time.*"

These were the goals – currently distant and remote.

The nurse smiled at my mother and left. Mom began to fade. I continued reading. The prognosis, the report went on, was "fair." The tentative duration of treatment was "30 days." After that, no one knew. Perhaps, the nursing home.

My mother did not seem perturbed; in fact, she was remarkably calm. She rested, eyes closed. I sat with her a while and reminisced. I was very tired, the weight of my mother's illness falling heavily upon me. It was an unexpected memory . . .

It was a warm, sunny day in September, and we had just started the school year. I was in the first grade at PS 44, "Admiral David Farragut Public School," named after the Civil War naval hero, on Prospect Avenue, and we were going on a class trip – a walk around the neighborhood. The teacher, Mrs. Nash, was a grandmotherly type with silver hair pulled back, a white blouse, and a black skirt down to her ankles. She was busily arranging the boys and girls by size in two separate parallel lines.

We assembled outside the classroom and walked down the stairs of the school. Mrs. Nash told us we were going on a walk through Crotona Park. I was excited because it was where my mother and I went for walks. We would pass Indian Lake, sliding rock, the baseball fields, and playgrounds, all my favorite places.

A mother of one of the kids from the class was there to help, a "teacher's aide" they called her, and she was nice. She told us to keep up, not to straggle. We walked through the gate leading into the park, past the ball fields and basketball courts, to Indian Lake. We saw two old men in a rowboat, fishing. There was a concession stand and Mrs. Nash bought each of us a snack. We sat down by the edge of the lake, talking, pointing at the old men in the boat, as they cast their lines, enjoying the warmth of the day. We went along a trail past the handball courts on one side and a patch of forest with bushes and large boulders on the other. There were squirrels and chipmunks scurrying about, and birds chirping.

Then we walked towards our park, the one across the street from my building. I did not realize we would walk this way. This was odd to me. School was where I went when I was not home and going past my house with my class seemed unusual, an unlikely pairing of two different worlds. One was a place of learning, discipline, and authority; the other, my home, a place of laughter, play, and affection. Merging the two, even briefly, seemed, to my young mind, not just implausible but incredible.

First, we walked up the hill to an oval sport area everyone called the "plateau," where my brothers and I played stickball. From there you could look down and see my house. I pointed it out to my classmates and to the aide who came over to see why I was so excited. I saw the tree-lined streets, the red brick building with the stone lions in front, and the fire escapes and clotheslines with laundry hanging. In the park across the street, there were benches with mothers and their children, the sandbox, swings, slides, and fountains, where I played. I told everyone that was my park and across the street was my house. The other kids nodded and asked me if I really lived here and was this really my park and if they could come and play. Mrs. Nash and the aide smiled and told us gently to move along.

We walked through the grass, down from the plateau, past another gate and into my park.

Then I saw a group of mothers with strollers and little children. The mothers were sitting on the wooden benches, conversing or laughing with one another, feeding their babies or watching over them. I recognized one of the kids, a chubby one with black hair, dungarees, and sneakers. It was Cliff. He was playing with a toy. I was beside myself with excitement. I told everyone he was my brother and everyone looked. Mrs. Nash smiled and said, "Ok, Rick, keep in line." But I shouted, unable to contain myself, "Hey, Cliff," I yelled, "come here!" Cliff looked around at the sound of the familiar voice and saw me. He smiled broadly, stood up and waved his hand. Then he ran over, pushing everyone aside to be with me. I put my arm over his shoulder, and we walked together. The aide said, "He looks just like you."

Then I saw a woman standing in the middle of the group of mothers who were chatting on the benches. She wore a blue dress and a red silk scarf. Her back was toward me. She had dark full hair, and when she turned, I saw she was my mother. I thought how beautiful she looked, like a dream or a movie, and how amazed and elated I was. I waved wildly, elbowing Cliff, pushing the other kids, saying, "That's my Mom, that's my Mom!" Then I yelled to her, "Hey, Mom!"

She heard my shouts, looked up, and a smile swept across her face, her teeth white and full, as she waved back. Cliff ran to join her, and I wanted to leave the line, leave my class, like Cliff, to be with my mother, but this was school and I could not; but I kept waving and smiling. I felt supremely happy. My mother was luminous and buoyant. She was not worried. She beamed at her five-year-old son, radiant like a goddess, flying toward me with passion and affection, an angel of mercy, of goodness and light, and the encounter and memory were sublime. She held Cliff, and they watched me walk off with my class, bidding farewell. I felt older, as if I were doing man's work, going off to school while Mom stayed home with Cliff.

"See ya, Ma," I said proudly, and the sense of joy was transcendent, my world at peace, as if God Himself had descended to prepare this revelation and bring me to the splendor and knowledge of pure love. I have never forgotten that moment.

I did not disturb my sleeping mother. Instead, I kissed her and returned home, remembering that image of my enchanted, youthful mother as lovely as could be.

-17-

My brother Cliff called from Brooklyn. "So, how's she doin'?" he asked impatiently.

"She's OK. She's not doing well from her stroke, but she's stable. Her heart and vital signs are OK. But she can't move her left side."

"She's still paralyzed?"

"Yeah, the entire left side. She can't get up or move. Can't eat. She's got an NG tube."

"Can't get outta bed?" he asked.

"No. She's bedridden."

"She must be goin' nuts."

"You would think so, knowing her," I said.

"No explanation for this? She was always so healthy, like a freakin' bull."

"Usual things. Her cholesterol, some sugar, and she's 78."

"Yeah, but she was so healthy before – like a bull."

"I know," I said.

"Really sucks. I'm so glad I had her over my house the day before she left. She had a good time. I still can't believe it. She was strong as a horse."

"It's a shock."

"And 'dis crap can happen jus' like that?" he asked.

"We've been through this, Cliff."

"You sure you didn't screw sumptin' up?"

"Ya gonna be a jerk?"

He backed off. "She goin' crazy?"

"No, she's been pretty calm."

"She's alert and everything?"

"She sleeps a lot, but when she's awake, she's alert, knows where she is."

"And she ain't depressed?"

"She doesn't seem to be, she seems tranquil."

"Can't believe it, I thought she'd be goin' outta her mind with this crap, I know I would . . . especially Ma, she's never been too calm."

"She's sleeping most of the time, but it's funny, how she's taking it," I said.

"So she's stable?"

"Yeah. You coming out this weekend?"

"Yeah, we'll all be out," Cliff said.

"Who's coming?"

"Me, Bloat, and Bones. Gums says he can't make it, the chump, he'll be out later." "Bloat" was Jerry, "Bones" was Jack, and "Gums" was Larry. And I was "Fatboy" or "Chubs." All names from the old days, garnered through the years, for various reasons, generally anatomic in nature, most no longer appropriate, but they persisted.

"So it took Mom having a stroke to get you jerks out here," I said.

"Hey, we're busy, man."

"Yeah."

"I still can't believe dis crap."

I had not told him anything about the TPA issue but thought he deserved to know. "There were some irregularities in her care," I said hesitantly.

"Whut's dat supposed ta mean?"

"There's a medicine she could have been given that might have helped."

"Like what!"

"I'll explain when you get here."

"Ah, crap!"

Dead Man's Hill was what we called it, the steep hill that ran from Crotona Park North to Boston Road, past the "El" on 174th Street, in the Bronx, two blocks from our house, where the kids went sleigh riding in the winter. There was an iron fence at the bottom of the hill, and Mom always warned me not to go down the hill. "You're too young, Rick," she said. "When you get older you can go." She told Jack and Jerry not to let me go down that hill. They said "Ok, Ma," and we put our coats and boots on and grabbed the sleds.

When we got there, there were a bunch of kids playing, making snowmen, throwing snowballs, and sleigh riding. "Don't go down that hill, heah?" Mom warned again. "I'll be back in an hour. I'm gonna get some groceries and visit Nona and Aunt Sophie." She left with Cliff in the stroller.

When we walked into the park, Jack and Jerry ran off to go sleigh riding. I played by myself in the snow. I watched the kids sleigh riding. Some of them did not look much older than me. Sheldon Schindler was there. He came running up with his sled, out of breath. He asked me why I wasn't sledding. I told him I was too young. His father was with him. He said, "You'll be alright, kid, I'll keep an eye on ya."

"My mother told me not to."

"I'll watchya, don't worry 'bout it. Sheldon's your age, just a little older, but close enough."

"I can't."

"Ya sure? Y'know we gotta a mattress down there ta cover the iron fence."

"No, that's OK, my Ma said no."

"Ok, kid, suit yourself . . ."

I walked over to the top of the hill. Jack and Jerry were waiting for me. "You heard what Mom said," Jack reminded me.

"Yeah, but what about the mattress and Mr. Schindler?"

"Sorry, Mom said no!"

So, Jack took his sled and went down the hill; he jumped off right before he got to the iron fence, and his sled slammed into the mattress. Then Jerry took his sled. He jumped off right before the iron fence, too. Then Sheldon went. And a bunch of other kids went. Some of them looked the same age as me. I took my sled and jumped on before Jack or Jerry got to the top. I rode past Jack, and he yelled, "Jump off the sled, you idiot!" I raced past Jerry, and he yelled, "Hey, Rick, you moron, jump off. Mr. Schindler was talking to someone. He turned and yelled, "Hey, Rick, jump off da sled!" But I kept going. Then, I hit a bump. I went sailing, over the mattress, like a bird, and into the iron fence at the bottom of Dead Man's Hill.

I heard a dull sound. Then my ears began to ring, and my head felt large. I rolled off the sled and lay on the ground. I felt something warm and sticky running down my face. I tried to get up. I noticed people running and shouting. I heard Mr. Schindler say, "Holy crap, kid, didn't no one tellya ta jump off da sled!" He climbed over the fence and ran to me. Jerry and Jack ran over. Jack told Jerry to call Mom. "Crap, Rick," Jack said, "we're dead now."

There was a crowd around me. Mr. Schindler picked me up. He wiped my face and I saw red stuff on his gloves. "What's that?" I asked. "It's blood, kid." I could see his face, but it was fuzzy. I felt the blood running down my face. I wanted to sleep, but Mr. Schindler wouldn't let me.

"Hey, kid, whatchya doin'?" he said, shaking me.

"Nothing," I mumbled, before drifting off again.

"Kid, don't do dis ta me!" He ran to the fence and handed me to someone on the other side. "Call an ambulance!" he yelled.

There was a small commotion. I heard someone shoving and jostling others. Jerry yelled, "No, Ma, no." Smack! I heard, and then another smack! "It wasn't my -"

"Shuddup, you idiot!" I heard my mother scream.

Then Jack said, "I told him not to –" Smack!

"Didn't I tell you not to let him go down that damn hill?"

The crowd parted, and I saw my mother bursting forth in a rage but also full of fear and worry. She ran to me. "Ricky," she cried, and she took me from Mr. Schindler, embracing me, as if to shield or protect me. She was crying.

"I'm sorry, Mrs. Moss," Mr. Schindler said. Mom kissed me and cradled me.

"Ricky, are you OK?" she pleaded. I didn't know if I was OK, but I liked my mother holding and kissing me. I closed my eyes and Mom screamed. "Rick!" And I opened them momentarily. "Don't do that, Rick, don't go to sleep!" she said desperately, afraid that perhaps I would not awaken. And I heard her weeping.

There was a siren. Mr. Schindler ran into the street and called the ambulance over. The drivers opened the back doors, and Mom carried me in. Mr. Schindler jumped in, the doors closed, and we raced down Boston Road, the siren blaring. Mom held me with one hand and the rail with the other, keeping us from falling with the sudden stops and turns. I lay there in her arms and heard Mom whimpering, "God help us, oh, dear God."

We drove to Fordham Hospital, right near the Bronx Zoo, and Mom carried me through the swinging doors. There were attendants in white uniforms, and Mom pleaded with them to hurry. Two aides in white coats placed me on a stretcher and brought me to a room. A doctor examined me. He shined a light in my eyes. He told me to stick my tongue out and close my eyes. Then he asked me to grab his hand and to wiggle my toes, which I thought was silly.

"He'll need an X-ray," he said. Mom was still crying. She pressed her pretty scarf against my head where it was bleeding.

They carried me into a large, dark room and placed me on a table. They shifted the X-ray machine hanging from the ceiling directly over my head. The table was cold. Everyone left when ordered to go behind a wall, including my mother who at first tried to stay. I wasn't frightened; rather I was mesmerized. Someone yelled, "Don't move." I heard strange, metallic sounds, and someone said, "OK."

The lights abruptly went on and normalcy seemed to return as people streamed back into the room. Someone took the film cartridge from beneath the table under my head. Mom waited with me. The doctor came in moments later and announced, "There's no fracture or internal bleeding. He should be fine."

"Oh, thank God," Mom cried.

We went back on the stretcher to the first room and someone stitched my head. I felt every one of those stitches and cried until he was done. Mom held me, putting her head to my chest, saying, "You're OK, son, you're OK."

I went home with Mom and was a hero. Everyone wanted to see the stitches. Mom forgave Jack and Jerry, but I never went sleigh riding down Dead Man's Hill again.

As I remembered this, I wondered what awaited my mother.

-18-

I caught up with Bruce Regan, Mom's internist, on the floor. I had not seen him in a couple of days.

"Hi, Rick," he said, businesslike, "I'm gonna get your Mom evaluated by the social worker for the skilled care unit."

"How long do you think she'll need in skilled care?"

"It depends on how she progresses." His manner seemed abrupt.

"Then what?"

"It just depends."

"What do you think about her condition?"

"She's dense," he said.

"You think I'll be able to take her home?"

"We have to see. It'll be hard to manage her at home if she doesn't improve."

"If I could get her to stand up and pivot, it would be all right."

"It's possible, we just have to see. It depends on the rehab. It'll take time."

"When will she go up to skilled care?"

"In a few days. I want her on the regular floor a while to make sure she's stable."

Judaism had always been at the center of my mother's life for she loved her faith. She sought to make it the center of our lives, too, although this was not easy. But we stud-

ied Hebrew, went to temple, and followed the holidays, as she demanded. Still, the world around us was changing and becoming more secular and its influences intruded into our cloistered province on Crotona Park North. In those early days, amidst the troubles, though, Mom did not abandon her faith. Rather, she clung more tightly, and so, in each of our own ways, did we.

Friday night was Sabbath night, the beginning of Shabbat, the day of rest, which coincided with the setting of the sun; it was that singular time each week that my mother had marked in earnest, observing the mitzvah (commandment) of keeping the Sabbath holy. We were not strict Jews, did not keep a kosher home or follow many of the Jewish Halacha or laws, but the ritual of greeting the Sabbath, my mother did not miss. As the sun dipped towards the horizon each Friday evening, the family gathered in the kitchen around the Sabbath table.

She set the special tablecloth, the Challah bread, the glass of wine, and the candles, all before the sun met the horizon. She placed a covering upon her head, lit the candles, and placed her hands over her face as she prayed quietly to herself. My mother's intensity always struck me, even as a child, with her eyes closed, her lips moving solemnly, mouthing the blessings silently, praying fervently, asking for blessings upon her children, family, and Israel, the light of the flames of the candles dancing across her face, onto the walls of our small kitchen, creating shadows. We did not move, none of us, an uncommon event, as if transfixed, as if instinctively acknowledging her devotion, and the sense of being in the presence of something holy. Mom had told us of the great Queen, Shabbat, the beautiful and bejeweled bride, and her groom, the people of Israel, and I wondered if this mythical goddess would enter our home, surrounded by angel emissaries, bestowing blessings, gifts, and remembrances.

"Praised art Thou, O Lord, King of the Universe," she recited in Hebrew, "You hallow us with mitzvot (command-

*ments) and command us to kindle the Sabbath lights." Thus,
the Sabbath began.*

*Mom would ask one of us to explain the Sabbath, its
meaning, and one of us would dutifully respond, "God created the world in six days, and on the seventh day He rested."*

*"Good," she would say, beaming, her spirit light and
merry. "Continue," she would say.*

*"God commanded us to rest on the seventh day, the Sab-
bath day, and to keep it holy."*

"Well done," she would say, smiling exultantly.

*Mom had taught us that the Sabbath was an island in
time, an oasis of peace, a sanctuary for rest and communion.
She explained (in unusually metaphorical language) that at
the instant of Shabbat, a door opened. Through this door, not
only could one peer back to the beginning of time when the
world was fresh and new, to the instant of the very first Sabbath when God rested after creating the world, but also ahead
to the Messianic age, when the Messiah would appear and
usher in God's Kingdom on earth. At this time, she said, all
would be tranquil and serene, all would worship the Lord, all
would be eternal Shabbat.*

*She dressed herself lovingly in this belief, adorned herself
happily in its transforming embrace; it buoyed and exhilarated her; she danced heartily in its richness and treasure,*

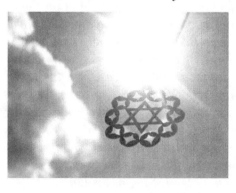 *and her devotion
to the tradition
flowed from her to
all of us, we, who
remained mesmer-
ized by her reverie
and inward jour-
ney. We listened
silently until she
intimated that we
could move and*

*speak, and the spell lingered as we completed the Sabbath
ceremony.*

-19-

I went to see my mother after office hours. I walked in just as the nurse was giving her a shot. "What's that?" I asked.

"Insulin, Dr. Moss," she answered. She wiped my mother's left thigh, the thigh that was completely numb, with an alcohol pad, and then administered the medicine through a tuberculin syringe. My mother felt nothing - a small consolation, I supposed, for having a stroke. The nurse withdrew the syringe, and held some pressure on the site.

"How much is she getting?"

"Ten units."

She had been on glyburide, an oral medicine for mild diabetes, before. "When did she start insulin?"

"Yesterday. Her sugars have been running a little high. She can probably get back on the glyburide when she can swallow again."

She had the nasogastric tube placed a couple days ago. I also noticed a clear plastic bag with a long silastic tube running alongside her leg hanging from the rail of the bed. "When did you place the catheter?" I asked.

"Yesterday. She's incontinent. Much easier this way, less skin breakdown."

"How long will she need that?"

"I don't know, Dr. Moss. It depends on how she progresses."

"She on antibiotics?"

"Yes, Cipro, 200 mg, every other day, IV."

"And Dr. Regan stopped the heparin drip?"

"Yes, she gets 5000 units sub-q, twice a day now."

"And aspirin."

"325 mg, once a day."

"By mouth?"

"Suppository."

Such were the changes after a stroke. An IV, NG tube, Foley catheter, suppositories, nothing by mouth, incontinent, unable to stand, walk, or feed oneself. Numb. Paralyzed. Utterly dependent. And a mere ten days before, she was taking walks and playing with her grandkids.

"Thanks."

She left the room.

I looked at my mother.

She shrugged.

"You feeling OK?" I asked.

"O-chhay." A couple of thickly slurred syllables were all. Still too weak to manage a subject pronoun. And she completely neglected her left side. She kept her head turned to the right, looked to the right, recognized sensory information coming only from the right. As if she was trying to withdraw from the left half of her body and, perhaps, the left side of the world. A reaction of anger and remorse? I wondered if she was even aware of it.

"Look over here, Ma," I said, holding my finger over to the left, trying to get her to swing her head. She tried to follow, reached the midline, and then stopped, wanting no part of it, wishing, perhaps, it would go away.

I looked at the collection of flowers, balloons, fruit baskets, and cards assembled on the counter by the window in her room, mostly from New York, but from well-wishers here in Indiana, too. "See the balloon and card from the kids? They wrote it themselves." I opened up the card and showed it to her. It was a handwritten thing with crayon drawings of a house and tree with a bunch of hearts, and their signatures. She seemed to smile at this. I looked at the names of the other cards. "And from Uncle Morris, Aunt Annie, Aunt Sophie." I rummaged around some more. "Uncle Willy, cousin Merilee, Stanley, Bobbie." She smiled again.

"I've got some good news for you, Ma," I said. "The boys will be here tonight." This was something of a bombshell. "They're flying in from New York, landing in Louisville, renting a car. Cliff, Jerry, and Jack."

She looked at me again as if to say, "Really?"

"Larry couldn't make it. He said he'd come out later. But, the rest of them will be here tonight."

And she smiled again, and then she gave me a look, which seemed to say, "Tell them not to bother." The proverbial Jewish martyr.

I was happy that my brothers were coming. Happy to share some of the burden. It was a strange coincidence that this had happened while Mom was visiting, but, since it had, it presented logistical problems for the family since no one else could easily visit her. This meant that the onus of tending to Mom fell to me, and it would be good to have someone else around to visit her, make her laugh, and act like the village idiots she always claimed we were. There was a higher grade of lunacy when we were all together, more than any of us could muster alone, a certain synergistic madness that crescendoed when we hit a critical mass, and both my mother and I could use a little of that.

When I opened the door to my home that evening, I heard a familiar voice: "Hey, yo, Chubs, whussup?"

"Who's that?" I answered back.

"Cool Breeze, man."

"Hey, yo, Breeze, whus happenin'?" I said in my thickest ghetto accent. I was glad to see that he was in a good mood.

"Fat boy . . ." Jerry chimed in, using another of my childhood nicknames.

"Hey Rick, how's it going?" Jack said.

And there they were, three out of the four brothers, like visions from the past, greeting me like nothing had changed, like we were still back home in our little two bedroom apartment in the Bronx. I was happy to see the maniacs, happy to see them here in Indiana. We drove over to the hospital. We got off the elevator on the third floor and walked down the corridor to Mom's room. As we approached the room, I sensed some hesitation in my brothers, a little uncertainty in their step, as if they were wondering how she would be, how she might look, unaccustomed as they were to seeing their mother ill. I entered the room first. I opened the curtains around her bed and was surprised to find her alert with eyes wide open.

"Hi, Momma, how are ya? Guess who's here?" The brothers promptly piled in, and for the first time since the stroke, she looked happy. She smiled in that crooked sort of way – her left facial paralysis commandeering her face – and gazed at the bouquet of familiar faces surrounding her.

I noticed, also, that since she had such difficulty speaking, she had adapted other forms of communication, most conspicuously the use of her right eye and eyebrow. She would open her right eye wide, raise her eyebrow, or tilt her head ever so slightly, all serving to convey an array of emotions and sentiments.

I was on her right, the side she favored. I asked Mom if she knew who I was, motivating her through my question, to speak. She gave me an annoyed look. "Go ahead, Mom, speak up, let me hear."

"Ricchh-y," she said, managing to convey through the slurred speech a trace of irritation.

"Your sons are here. Are you happy?" And she nodded and smiled, appearing quite pleased. I could not help but notice how much their presence here was helping *me*, as if the emotional burden of Mom's illness had been suddenly split four ways.

I shifted her head so she could better see her other sons. She smiled. No words, but a nice smile. Her right eyebrow went up, and then the crooked half smile.

The brothers seemed to have loosened up a little as they acclimated to the sight of their disabled mother.

"Hey, Ma, howyadoin', yaw gonna be fine," Cliff said, the thick New York brogue bouncing around the room like a ball, sounding odd in this milieu. The boys in general were already quite a sight here in this tiny burg in rural Indiana. They were so loud and boisterous, even just getting out of the elevator and walking through the halls.

Mom was perking up for the first time since it had all happened. And the inevitable jokes and gags soon followed. This was standard for the brothers, for whom circumstances were irrelevant. It could have been a funeral. I decided to leave them alone with her, feeling they would be more at ease if I were gone. I took my kids downstairs. We returned about a half hour later. The brothers and Mom remained in good spirits. When it was time to go, I lined Arielle and Noah alongside Mom's bed. They each held her hand. Mom's eyes lit up. It was beautiful to see how radiant she became in the presence of her grandchildren. The kids kissed her and bowed as my wife had taught them, Thai-style. We left the hospital and returned home, noisy as ever.

The children were sleeping and Jack and Jerry had retired to their rooms. I was standing alone in the backyard, listening to the sounds of the forest when Cliff came out. It had thus far been a pleasant time with my brothers.

"So what were these irregularities you were talkin' about?" he asked.

"There's a blood thinner they use for stroke patients that might have helped. It's called TPA. She never got it."

"Why da hell not?" he said, folding his arms across
his chest.

"The medicine has to be given within three hours of
the stroke," I said. "Past that and it can cause bleeding.
I wasn't sure when she had the stroke."

"But didn't you see her? You were wit' her, you told
me."

"There were three hours before the stroke when I
wasn't with her. But I saw her walk out, that's right."

"Isn't dat when she had it?"

"I couldn't be certain."

"But you saw her walk out!"

"I wasn't sure."

He looked away angrily.

"Why didn't you tell 'em, so she coulda gotten da
frickin' medicine?"

"I didn't know!"

"Whaddaya mean ya didn't know? Whaddayou, a
frickin' screwball?

I turned away.

"You're a big important doctor, right? Dat's when
she had da stroke. Rick, whattsamatta wit you?

"Alright, already!"

"You screwed dis up, Rick," he said disgustedly.
"Now she's an invalid."

-20-

Patoka Lake was the largest lake in Indiana, formed by a dam built some thirty years ago on the Patoka River by the Army Corp of Engineers to prevent the yearly floods that river regularly visited upon the inhabitants of the surrounding lowlands. In so doing, it created a beautiful lake, enclosed by forested hills that made one think of nothing so much as a Greek Island in the Mediterranean Sea.

It was, in a word, stunning, which was unusual, because Indiana was generally not a "stunning" state. It had rolling hills, emerald and brown fields of corn and wheat, grassy meadows, white picket fences, and barns and silos poised like monuments amidst waves of shimmering, tasseled corn, all quite splendid really but not "stunning," say, in the manner of the Rocky Mountains or the California coast. Rather, it was rural Indiana, Middle America, with timeless, melodic rhythms, pauses and silences, the quiet transition of the days and seasons, tranquil, soothing, and ordinary, but lovely and pleasing just the same.

But one came to appreciate southern Indiana with its simple beauty, the unassuming manner of its people, their basic decency and friendliness, their well-honed virtues of hard work and self-reliance on quiet display. It was folksy and, perhaps, corny, but not flamboyant. They were not cowboys or cattle rustlers and certainly not large urban dwellers, but farmers and factory workers. They were not rich and may even be poor, but generally they possessed of a quiet dignity. They did not rush too much, nor did they fuss, and they were possessed of fewer emotional emergencies. The land and its people were well suited for each other, as if the calming qualities of the land had rubbed off on its inhabitants.

It was also the ancestral home of my mother, the place where she returned to be with her son, the doctor, the wanderer, to take ill. It was logical to reunite with me here, in the land where she was born and remembered fondly. She was one of nine children, Sephardic Jews from the village of Monastir in Macedonia, formerly part of the Turkish Empire. Mom was the sixth child of Jacob and Rebecca Camhe, born in Indianapolis, Indiana, a single generation removed from the motherland.

But today was about Patoka, the beautiful lake that transcended its state, eclipsed the quiet, pastoral countryside from which it arose, a majestic and magnificent by-product of man's need to recontour nature to suit his needs, in this case, to damn the floodwaters of the Patoka river. Patoka Lake was brilliant, its smooth waters glistening in the Indiana sun, cradled by densely wooded hills, embraced by a sapphire sky, only occasionally accented by tufts of cottony cloud.

It was a day of laughter for the family, which, under the circumstances, was remarkable, a testimonial to the restorative power of this magical lake, named after an Indian tribe that lived here centuries ago. Out of illness could come health, out of sadness could come joy, out of tragedy, some form of redemption; and on this summer day, with the family brought together because of a tragedy, we managed to laugh and be happy.

Cliff and Jerry rented a motorboat from Patoka Lake Marina and my two kids and I joined them. We sliced through rippled waters, explored coves, drifted into lagoons, cruised past land's edge watching branches and birds dart by, hurtling headlong across the lucid expanses. It was hearty fun, and the kids were in their element, giddy with laughter, as the boat churned and galloped across the great lake. There was only the moment, the eternal now, and the family was united, our thoughts and energies consumed for the time by our watery antics, plowing the watery lanes on a cloud of foam, leaving waves in our wake.

We anchored the boat in the middle of the lake. Noah, the wild one all of three years, insisted on diving off the rail like his uncle Cliff. He was nimble, graceful even, for so young an age. A natural athlete, he exuded physical confidence, his body poised and quick, like a young cougar. I held his hand as he stood on the rail and plunged headlong into the water. He acted as if injuring himself were outside the realm of possibility, as if fear did not exist.

Arielle, age six, on the other hand, was his opposite; she was gentle and demure. She descended the ladder on the side of the boat, daintily sampling the water with her toes, making sure of the temperature, and only then, after much contemplation, immersing herself into it inch by inch. She was already a "lady," in the old-fashioned sense: soft-spoken, reticent, loath to draw attention to herself, but with keen intelligence and precocious wit, an American daughter imbued with Asian manners. She was as graceful in her restraint as Noah was in his athletic abandon.

The sun dropped in the sky, creating a soft, luminous light on Patoka Lake, and promising a spectacular sunset, my mother's kind of sunset. Jerry was helping Noah bait a hook.

"Uncle Jerry," I heard Noah's voice, "can we go fishing again tomorrow?" Uncle Jerry smiled and patted his nephew on the head affectionately.

"Sure," he answered.

But the weight of my mother's illness was not distant. It was close, a clandestine presence, invisible but palpable, exerting its effect; a force concealed only marginally by the enchantments of the day. I drove the van home, Cliff in the passenger seat beside me. The kids were quiet in the back, tired, and Jerry was beginning to fall asleep. He looked old as he drifted off. Cliff and I sat silently at first. He shifted nervously before finally speaking. I felt the familiar indignation present in his voice, and, perhaps, a touch of the ancient jealousies. He had said nothing since our conversation the first night, but I could see he was frustrated.

"So what's up wit' Ma?" he said in a tone I did not like. Our last discussion had dredged up all the negative emotions and self-hatred that I had been desperately running from.

"You want to go through this again?" I said.

"Is she gonna get better?"

"I don't know," I answered.

"What do the doctors say?"

"It's gonna take time."

"You mean she's gonna stay like dis?"

"I don't know!"

"Same crap! Meanwhile, she's lyin' in a frickin' bed."

"I can't make her stand up and walk."

"I don't want her in no nursing home."

"Neither do I."

"You can't take care of her like dis."

"I know!"

"Always so smart," he said, turning toward the passenger window.

He deliberately did not bring up the "irregularities" we had discussed earlier, for which I was grateful.

I heard Jerry stirring as the unhappy exchange ended. It became suddenly quiet, both of us feeling foolish.

"Take it easy, Cliff," Jerry said. "Rick's doing what he can. It's nobody's fault." And with these words, a troubled silence returned. I looked at Cliff. He turned away, muttering. Then Jerry started up again but on a different tack. Instead, he gave expert testimony about hunting bear in Montana and shooting elk in Canada, about a redneck hunting guide he had in West Virginia, about nearly drowning in an icy stream in Idaho, about tracking wild boar in Florida, about the joys of venison, and the advantages of a cross bow. Noah was enthralled and everyone relaxed.

On Sunday morning, Cliff and Jerry got up early for a couple rounds of golf, and then went over with Jack to visit Mom. I did not join them. I knew that this short bubble of time with the brothers would soon end, and that I would be alone with her again. When the brothers finished their visit, they returned to my house for lunch.

Afterwards, we discussed some unpleasantries, issues we had always avoided, but now, with Mom's illness, could ignore no longer. The major concerns were power-of-attorney, the use of advanced life support, nursing home arrangements, and what to do with Mom's apartment and assets. Jerry had brought these questions up before, particularly the nursing home question, but we had deferred them. It was something on the order of discussing family cemetery plots, an unhappy consideration however legitimate.

As a physician and the one immediately involved in overseeing her care, I recommended that I have power-of-attorney. Cliff agreed immediately, which surprised me. I sensed hesitation from Jerry. Perhaps, he felt I was usurping his traditional role, he who had watched over her finances for the last decade. That I was a physician did not automatically qualify me, and perhaps he resented the assumption that it did. Was a doctor better qualified than a non-physician to direct the care of a loved one? Not necessarily, but there was that undercurrent of thought in the family, and he rebelled against it.

The decision actually was not medical but moral, and who was best suited to pursue Mom's interests. Being a physician was to my advantage, but the main factor was my proximity. Other than that, any of my brothers would have been valid choices.

I looked at Jerry. I sensed he wanted to contest it, but felt ridiculous doing so. He agonized briefly but finally assented, albeit begrudgingly, as if to imply he really did not favor the choice. He grunted something about speaking with his lawyer to make arrangements. He insisted, perhaps resentfully, that the brothers be contacted for anything significant. This, of course, was not a question.

On the question of advanced life support or resuscitative measures, I felt that at this stage, Mom should have everything medicine could offer. There was nothing in her overall condition or mental status that suggested her life was no longer worth living. Despite everything, she could think, smile, recognize her grandchildren, and, hence, experience joy and pleasure. No one disagreed, nor did I expect anyone to. This was straightforward.

Regarding her apartment, it was still too early to say. No one knew if she would ever return to it, but we agreed that we would maintain it in the meantime. The final point, regarding a nursing home, would be decided later. Jerry seemed anxious to discuss it now, but there was little appetite for it by anyone else, and so we deferred it.

I noticed that Cliff seemed morose, his combativeness displaced by an uncharacteristic melancholy. No such gloom infected Jerry. Having completed the objectionable tasks, he immediately shifted gears, becoming jovial and blustery, a personality adaptation completely at odds with the somber qualities he had growing up in the Bronx. It grew out of a successful twenty-year experience in selling life insurance. But while he could be very friendly and supportive, he could also turn quickly and become bellicose, particularly with me.

With Jack, it all depended. He hovered between dark depression on the one hand and contentious assertiveness on the other, contingent on the whim of his prevailing mood and the effects of the various medicines he took. Today, he was rambunctious and high-spirited. I noticed that neither of them seemed overly anxious about Mom.

Cliff, as quarrelsome as he had been, seemed more concerned for his mother, her tragedy visibly affecting him. Recognizing this, I was more tolerant of his hostility. I did not doubt the concern of my other brothers for their mother, but I felt the two youngest, Cliff and I, had formed the strongest bonds with her.

With the main issues decided, we enjoyed a final lunch together. We embraced and bid farewell. My brothers piled into their rented car and drove off to the airport to catch their plane back to New York. Cliff was already making plans to return in a couple of weeks with his kids, his anger, it seemed, abated. Before leaving, he told me to do everything I could. I assured him I would.

The skilled care evaluation was straightforward: "Patient name: Matilda Moss.

Age: 78.

Physician: Bruce Regan.

Address: 510 Main Street, Roosevelt Island, New York, NY, 10044.

Pay Source: Medicare A and B. Insurance: Blue Cross out of Aetna.

Memorial Hospital admission date: September 5, 1998. Room 357.

History and Physical date: September 5, 1998. On chart: Yes."

Skilled Care was actually the fifth floor of Memorial Hospital. It was a way station between the acute, short-term care in a hospital and the long term chronic care of a nursing home.

I continued reading the report:

"Diagnosis: 1. Acute Cerebrovascular Accident (CVA) 2. Acute Left Hemi paralysis." There were others, but these were the main ones. She had diabetes, cholesterol, arthritis, even mild "cognitive decline" by history, but the first two were what had brought her to skilled care.

"Chest X-ray date: September 9. Chest X-ray clear of Tuberculosis: Yes. Allergies: none."

Then, very importantly: "Current therapy which meets criteria for skilled care:" These were listed in detail, but it was the first three that mattered most: "Physical therapy, occupational therapy, and speech therapy."

Thus began the campaign to encourage her limp left side to reassert itself. All the research, positive thoughts, and prayers were helpful (perhaps most to myself), but incidental to this: the dull, monotonous repetitions designed to engage the left side of her body. There were other items tossed in to meet admission criteria to assure reimbursement from the Medicare Gods - the nasogastric tube, the intravenous antibiotics, and so on, but it was the trinity of therapies that were the primary focus of her care.

I scanned quickly the remainder of the report:

"Elimination: catheter. Mobility: up in chair. Mental status: orientated. Activities of Daily Living" (ADLs). This asked how much of the ADLs did she require assistance with. The answer: "total care." Additional comments: "neuro checks and vital signs every four hours."

Then: "Qualified for skilled care: Yes."

There you had it. She had met the demands of the skilled care bureaucracy. Plans for transfer were underway, and soon she would have a temporary new home. At least she no longer required formal hospitalization. Skilled care was a thirty-day transitional unit to allow patients to establish whether they could regain sufficient autonomy and function to return home. And if unable – to be transferred to a nursing home for chronic long-term care.

I put down the chart and went into my mother's room, where I sat down beside her, the habit instantly familiar. There had been a four-day hiatus of such private moments at her bedside with my brothers visiting, but, with their departure, I quickly resumed the pattern. I felt alone beside her, more than before, a painful yearning usurping the more ordinary despair of yesterday. I was not consoled by anything, her calm, sleeping face, the ticking of the clock, the flowers, balloons, and get well cards pouring in from around the country, the pesky nurse peeking in. Everything seemed configured to annoy and harass me, to unsettle my perilous grasp of things, to uproot my inconsistencies.

I settled myself by gazing at her. A kind of meditation. She was resting, eyes closed, breathing deeply, her face smooth and pink. She did not rouse when I entered, and I did not disturb her. I would let her sleep, allow the healing of deep rest to rejuvenate her and hope for a reversal. I could imagine all this as a trivial illness, a bout with a virus or some other such nuisance, easily undone by a good night's slumber and a cup of tea. To that, I would add my own presence, returning the favor of a thousand such moments before when she stood vigil over me, wishing her well, hoping for a return to health, a recovery of her erstwhile faculties and powers. By so doing, I may alter the intermittent waves of aversion that assailed me.

As I sat next to her, I closed my eyes, and reminisced about the past, my internal derangements abating, the paradoxes dissipating, the vexations submerging out of mind. I drifted into another time, when I was young, my brothers were young, and we, all of us, were young.

It was the day of Jack's Bar Mitzvah. I was five. We were having the party at Aunt Sophie's apartment on Hoe Avenue with all the aunts, uncles, and cousins. Nono and Nona (my maternal grandparents) had nine kids. And their kids had kids. Mom had five kids, Aunt Annie had three kids, Uncle Morris had six kids, Uncle Paul had two kids, Aunt Rae had three kids, Aunt Sophie had two kids, and then there were second and third cousins from Nono and Nona's brothers and sisters, and from the husbands and wives of Mom's brothers and sisters, and then everyone's friends. It would be a festive occasion.

The brothers prepared for the event. We showered, brushed our teeth, and combed our hair. We shined our shoes and got our clothing ready. Mom ironed our shirts and cleaned the suit jackets that Aunt Sophie and Aunt Rae gave us, hand-me-downs from their kids. We put our little suit jackets on and strutted around proudly.

Because we were poor, we didn't have money to have a regular Bar Mitzvah with a rabbi at the synagogue. We were going to have it at Nono's apartment on Minford Place instead, with Nono presiding, and the reception after at Aunt Sophie's.

Nono had white hair and wrinkles and sat in a big chair in the living room in front of the TV and never moved or smiled. He never asked us how we were or if we wanted something to eat. He never even looked at us. We were afraid of Nono. Mom told us he was a Turk and that's how Turks were and that she was afraid of Nono, too. Everyone was afraid of Nono.

*When Mom and the five boys walked into Nono's house,
Jack instantly became fidgety. Jack was nervous in general.
He had pimples and slouched. He had a big nose, thick glasses, and was skinny. He was sullen and didn't talk. We were
worried that Jack would get nervous in front of Nono and not
read his Hebrew right.*

*We sat down in the living room. Jack was in his suit,
thirteen years old, the day of his Bar Mitzvah. It was supposed to be a celebration. This was the day he became a man.
Nono didn't say a word. He grumbled for Jack to stand beside
him. He brought out a brand new tallis (prayer shawl) for
Jack in honor of his Bar Mitzvah and placed it around his
shoulders. Then he rolled up Jack's left shirtsleeve. He recited
the blessings as he wrapped the tefillin (ritual prayer boxes
and straps) around his left arm and hand and the other piece
around his head. Jack squirmed.*

*The room was dark except for a candle. Nono began read-
ing from the prayer book in Hebrew, conducting his own service, which none of us understood. He closed his eyes and
prayed quietly. Then he put his prayer book down. He looked
up at the ceiling and rolled his eyes up into his head. He
raised his hands up in the air. He began singing, moving his
head back and forth with a crazy smile on his face. He began
skipping and spinning in circles. He danced around the dark
room, and we watched him, not saying a word.*

*Nono opened his eyes. He told Nona to get some wine.
Nono blessed it and drank it. Then he spread his tallis over
Jack's head and blessed him. Nono handed Jack the prayer
book and told him to read the sections he had prepared. Jack
mumbled a few words in Hebrew but then stopped. He looked
at the book and tried to read, but nothing came out. He managed another few squeaks in Hebrew but stopped again. He
kept glancing at the fingers of his left hand, where Nono
wrapped the tefillin. He complained they hurt and were
going numb. He groaned and seemed to be having trouble
breathing. He kept adjusting his collar and tie as if it were
too tight. He stretched his neck and cleared his throat. He*

wiped his brow. His eyes seemed to cross, and I thought he was going to pass out. Then he covered his mouth.

Nono asked Mom what he was doing. Mom said he was going to vomit. Nono looked at Jack in amazement. What's wrong with him? Jack didn't answer. He looked at the floor, avoiding his eyes, still covering his mouth. He began having dry heaves. Mom told him to run. Jack ran down the hallway, and about half way to the bathroom let out a loud belch and puked all over the floor. He fell to his hands and knees, still puking, his new tallis covered in it. Mom helped Jack up and got him into the bathroom. Nono yelled that it was a sin to bring the tallis and tefillin into the bathroom. We heard him barfing in the toilet.

A few minutes later, Mom walked Jack back into the living room where we were all waiting. He looked weak. He smelled. His eyes were glazed. None of us said anything. Mom kissed Jack and said proudly, "Congratulations, son, today you are a man." Nono didn't say a word.

After the service with Nono, Mom got sick. I never saw Mom sick before. I thought Mom couldn't get sick.

She had left earlier to go to Aunt Sophie's apartment to help prepare for Jack's party. When we arrived, Mom was lying on the couch. She had her dress on, high-heeled shoes, lip stick, eye shadow, and her hair was pulled up, but she was lying there, white as a sheet.

"I'm dying," I heard Mom say.

Jack and Larry wept. So did Aunt Sophie. Then Jerry started. Stanley and Bobby, Aunt Sophie's kids, began crying. Uncle Joe, Aunt Sophie's husband, with the big cigar that he always smoked, blinked and blew cigar smoke out through his nose. Uncle Morris and Aunt Libby walked in.

"Ah, Tilly, honey," Aunt Sophie said, "what's the matter?"

"I'm dying."

"Tilly, it's Jack's Bar Mitzvah."

"I can't breathe, Sophie."

"Oh, God," Aunt Sophie said.

"My chest, Sophie, I'm having a heart attack."

"You're strong as an ox, Tilly, there's nothing wrong with your heart."

"I've got chest pain," she gasped.

"But you never had trouble with your heart before."

"It's my heart, Sophie, I'm tellin' ya."

"Was it something she ate?" Aunt Annie asked.

"She hasn't eaten anything," Aunt Sophie said.

"What's the matter, Tilly," Uncle Joe said in a reassuring voice, trying to comfort her.

"I'm not gonna make it, Joe."

"Should I call the doctor, Tilly," Uncle Joe asked.

"She's having a heart attack, of course you should call the doctor," Aunt Annie said.

"No, Joe, don't bother, let me die in peace," Mom said.

"Call the doctor, he's down the block," Uncle Morris said,

"No Morris," Mom said.

"Shuddup, Tilly," Uncle Morris said.

Aunt Sophie got on the phone and called Doctor Pinski.

Then Aunt Rae walked in with her husband Artie and their three kids, Sylvia, Jerry, and Stevie. Aunt Rae was the oldest of the nine kids in Mom's family and the Queen Bee. When she spoke, everyone snapped.

"What's going on here?" she yelled.

"Tilly's dying," Aunt Annie blurted.

"Oh for cripe sakes, Tilly, what's the matter with you, you were fine an hour ago!" Aunt Rae said. Mom, who usually jumped when Aunt Rae said a word, didn't flinch. "I'll betchya it's that nogood husband of hers, leavin' her with five kids, that scoundrel, that fink, that mongrel from Brooklyn. It's no wonder. She must be a nervous wreck, poor thing."

Mom waved for Jack. "Come here, son," she said. Jack walked over in his clothes that still smelled of vomit.

"Yeah, Ma," he said shakily.

"Be good, son."

"I will, Ma."

"Try to remember your mother, son."

"I will, Ma."

"You're a man now, son."

"I know, Ma."

"I'm going, son."

Jack really blubbered now, kneeling in front of Mom, holding her hand.

He left Mom, still crying, and came over to me. *"If Mom dies,"* he said, *"I'm gonna kill you."*

"Why, what'd I do?" I said.

"You're always drivin' her crazy, runnin' around, and fighting with Cliff."

"Shuddup, Bones, I didn't do nothin'," I said. *"It's 'cause you're so skinny and have pimples and vomit all the time."*

When I heard Mom say she was dying, I got scared. I knew what death meant after the night of bloody murder and Linda. It meant I would never see her again or that she couldn't take me to Cheap Charlie's or buy me tootsie rolls. I didn't want Mom to have to go into the ground somewhere in a box with grass growing over her. I wanted her to stay right here, in the Bronx, with us kids, in Aunt Sophie's apartment for the party.

I walked up to Mom, crying. *"Mom,"* I said, *"I don't want you to die, we have to have Jack's party, and everyone's here, all the aunts and uncles and cousins and Nona and Nono. You can't die."* She barely opened her eyes to look at me.

"I can't make it, Ricky."

"Why, Ma? You were fine before. You're all dressed up and pretty. Why?"

"I'm sick, son." I placed my head against Mom's chest, crying, the whole family standing over us, staring in disbelief.

"O God in heaven," I heard the aunts say.

"I've got a picture I made for ya, Ma." I pulled a crumpled piece of paper out of my pocket with a drawing of a Jew-

ish star and a Torah. "See, Mom, I made it for ya. I'll be a
good Jew like you always wanted and sit still at synagogue
and not talk about Jesus."

She kept holding her chest, trying to breathe, but smiled
a little when I showed her the picture.

There was a knock on the door. Doctor Pinski walked in
with his black bag.

"Over here, Doc," Uncle Morris said, "she's on the
couch."

Doctor Pinski held Mom's hand and said, "Hi, Tilly, how
are you?" Mom shook her head. He seemed relaxed, which
made everyone feel better. He opened his black bag and pulled
out some doctor things. He listened to her chest, checked her
heart, and looked at her eyes and throat. He wrapped a black
bag around her arm and squeezed it, watching a little dial for
her blood pressure. Then he turned and said in a calm voice
that Mom was fine.

"Huh?" Uncle Morris said.

"She had a panic attack, nothing more. Probably stress
related. She has a lot on her mind."

"Ya kiddin' me doc?"

"No."

"What's she panicking for, the Bar Mitzvah's over?"

"That no good husband, that's what," Aunt Rae said.
"Five kids without a lousy dime to her name."

"Ah, for cryin' out loud, Tilly," Uncle Morris said. "All
right, Doc, can ya give her somethin' to settle her so we can
get the party started."

"She won't need to be hospitalized?" Aunt Annie asked.

"Are you outta your mind, Annie," Uncle Morris said.
"It's all in her head! She's a little crazy, that's all. She's fine!"

Everyone seemed to relax. Mom didn't seem any better,
though, just lying there, mumbling to herself. Doctor Pinski
pulled out one of those long needles and a syringe from his
bag and gave Mom a shot in the arm. Everyone else moved
into the living room. Uncle Joe started handing out cigars
and pouring drinks. Aunt Sophie told me what a beautiful

picture I made for Mom and how that was as important as the medicine Doc Pinski gave her. "Want some soda, honey," she said, pouring me a Dixie cup.

Uncle Joe turned on some Greek music, one of the family favorites. Uncle Paul began snapping his fingers, hopping, stooping, and scraping the floor with his hand, yelling "Ooompah," like Zorba the Greek. A dance line formed behind him, following him around the apartment, past Mom on the couch, through the kitchen, the bedrooms, the hallway, the foyer, and back into the living room. Uncle Willy and Aunt Esther were yelling from the street below to let them in.

"What goin' on up there, we've been ringing the doorbell for half an hour," Aunt Esther screamed. Uncle Joe opened the window and poured whiskey on them, yelling, "Yer sister Tilly scared the crap outta us, and now we're havin' a frickin' good time!" Uncle Joe grabbed Jack, smacking him in the back, pouring him a glass of whiskey. "C'mon, son," he said, "today you are a man!" And everyone guffawed.

Doctor Pinski put his things back in his black bag. Uncle Morris paid him, gave him a drink, and said, "Thanks, Doc, that was great, you saved the whole damn day."

Mom sat up suddenly, as if waking from a dream. She looked beautiful again, like a queen, with her red lips, her hair pulled up, and her sparkly gown. She walked into the living room. Her sisters Sophie, Annie, Rae, and Esther greeted her.

"Ya nearly gave us a heart attack, Tilly," Aunt Rae yelled. Everyone roared. They watched as Mom danced, clapping and hooting and encouraging her, she, smiling now, savoring the attention like a child. Uncle Morris licked a twenty-dollar bill and stuck it to her forehead. He did the "money dance," twirling around her, snapping his fingers. Mom closed her eyes and made circles, arms spread, in her own little world. Then Nona came up to Mom, kissed her on the cheek and planted a roll of bills in her hand. Mom opened her eyes, and kissed Nona, almost crying. Uncle Morris pushed Jack into the circle.

"*Get in dere wit' ya mudda,*" *he said. And the two, Mom and Jack, danced together, Jack awkward and self-conscious, and Mom still smiling at him, her second oldest, on his big day. Nono, the tough old Turk, never budged from his chair, watching everyone like a king, the aunts hanging over him like little bees, bringing him whiskey and food.*

I danced with Mom. All the boys danced with her. We ate, drank, and ran around in Aunt Sophie's apartment, crowded with relatives and friends for Jack's Bar Mitzvah. Everything was OK again, and Mom was OK, even without a husband or money and with five kids to feed.

-21-

I took the elevator to the fifth floor today to visit my mother in her new room in skilled care. It was in the hospital yet "outside" of it, treated as a separate part. Dr. Regan had formally discharged her and readmitted her to skilled care. This meant nothing more than getting in the elevator, going up a couple flights, and moving into a different bed. In the skilled unit, a physician was required to see his patient once a week, instead of daily, and the patient to nurse ratio was much higher. It was an indication, at least, that she had stabilized enough to be moved from the hospital. As far as her recovery from the stroke and return of function, it signified nothing.

I walked off the elevator with my white coat, shirt and tie, pressed trousers, leather shoes, and into the skilled care unit. Now I was only a family member visiting an ailing relation. I noticed there was a more relaxed atmosphere here than in the acute care section of the hospital, which made sense given that it was more of a chronic care facility. The mood was friendlier and less hectic, which, I imagined, was more soothing for the patients.

The nurse caring for my mother saw me and immediately stepped forward to give me an update. On the regular floor, it was often a chore to find the nurse caring for your patient, busy as they were scrambling from room to room, passing medicines, checking vital signs, admitting and discharging patients.

"Your Mom was really talking last night," she said almost excitedly.

"Really?" I said, surprised.

"Yes, she was talking up a storm."

"Still slurred?"

"Yes, but easy to understand."

"Is she eating?"

"Very little. She still needs the NG tube. But speech therapy is working with her."

She led me to Mom's room. She was in a deep sleep.

"She's tough to rouse in the morning," the nurse said. "But she perks up at night. Makes us all laugh. She's a doll."

I had never thought of Mom as a "doll." A character, yes, but not a doll.

I sat alongside her. "Momma, wake up," I said, stroking her forehead.

She roused slightly and opened her eyes. There was a brief moment of recognition, and then she was asleep again.

"She's tough in the morning, Dr. Moss, but come nighttime, she's as lively as can be. We're finding out all about you and your brothers, y'know, quite a lively crew she tells us." She chuckled slightly. "And she's so proud of you, Dr. Moss. You're special to her."

"Oh, really?" I said, appreciating her generous words.

"Oh, yeah, you're the apple of her eye," she said plainly. "And she was going on about Arielle. My goodness, how she loves that little girl – and the way she plays the violin!"

I remained by Mom's side for a while, beset by premonitions. The nurse seemed so bubbly and optimistic, the opposite of how I felt. I watched Mom, seeking consolation in her peaceful demeanor. Then I offered up a prayer, more for myself than anyone. Mom opened her eyes briefly before drifting off. I held her hand and kissed her.

It was strange having my mother in the hospital here in Jasper, Indiana, this tiny enclave in the rural Midwest. I was not from here, not one of the Jasper gentry whose families had been here for generations, since they founded the town more than a century ago. I was Jewish, from the Bronx, and married to an Asian woman. Between the two of us, we could not have stood out more. What saved us from internal exile was that I was a physician. There was still magic in that profession, and no matter my religious affiliation or place of origin, the community treated me respectfully. Still, that I was strange and different could not be denied. The Jewish part was probably most significant.

Although I never experienced bigotry, I suspected it may have been there under the surface, at least in some individuals. Most, however, seemed to find my religious background to be a point of interest, if not fascination. Indeed, I engaged in a variety of interfaith activities with local churches and spoke about my religion at some of the schools. And many religious Christians, I found, were strong supporters of Israel, which I appreciated. More importantly, though, were the social implications. Being Jewish meant that I did not belong to the local churches, that my wife did not join in the activities of Christian women's groups, and that my kids didn't go to Sunday school here in town.

But now, my mother was in the hospital, this beehive of activity, where babies were born, gallbladders snipped, and cancers diagnosed. In a way, I felt exposed, as if the founding principle of my life had been discovered. My mother was like a relic from my past, a living fossil, so to speak, holding insights and knowledge about me. She was an artifact that opened new doors and understanding about a lost epoch, my past and that of my family's. Now she was here amidst the denizens of southeastern Indiana, in Memorial Hospital in Jasper, who could glimpse her amused, intrigued, wondering about this strange woman from afar, with her curious accent and mannerisms, so different from the usual patrons.

For the first time, I felt as if my past, the essential facts of my early years, were open and accessible to those who had formerly known me only as "Dr. Moss." That bloodless, one-dimensional image now gave way to a more robust likeness that could be viewed from different angles, like a cubist painting. In my mother's presence, I took on color and perspective, definition, and character. She fleshed out the portrait, adding depth and resonance.

Now, I was a son, the fourth son in a family of five boys who grew up in the Bronx. This was startling new information. I had a mother who one could see, touch, and talk to, which implied, of course, that Dr. Moss had once been a boy, a mischievous little demon who ran around and got into fights. I acquired a past with layers, hidden niches, and back-story.

As some of the nurses gleefully recounted for me on my frequent visits, they had learned all about me - that I played shortstop, quarterback, and guard, rode a two-wheeler down the hill on Strong Street with Cliff sitting on the handlebars and my friend, Richie, on the rear fender.

Had they delved deeper, they may have learned that I poured water from the roof of my building onto pedestrians below or "itchy balls" at police cars (for which my mother was not pleased). I had "punching" contests with rivals from Marmion Avenue, broke windows at PS 86 playing stickball, and turned hydrants on in the summer. I drank chocolate egg creams for a dime at Schechter's and played "Ringoleevio" and "Johnny on the Pony" at PS 67. I went to Yankee Stadium religiously and papered my walls with newspaper clippings of Mickey Mantle. I had fistfights with Willie Mays devotees and annoying Met fans. I wore a Garrison belt and later carried a switchblade. I rode the subways with my pal, Johnnie, and was knifed, robbed, and had a gun held to my face.

My mother, perhaps, in her more lucid moments, told her nurses of her brood of five boys growing up in the Bronx or, perhaps, about her life as a little girl in a family of nine children growing up in Indianapolis. She wore her Jewish star proudly on her necklace, something that perhaps none of her caregivers had ever seen before. With my mother here, in other words, I took on nuances and depths hitherto unknown.

My mother was an open book about my past, in the way she looked, in what she said, in her memories of me growing up. In her being and manner, she defined who I was without saying a word. As source and repository of my history and that of my family's, she was sacred, like an ancient scripture or vessel.

She was the embodiment of our past,
custodian of the family record,
guardian of cryptic knowledge, curator of secrets,
someone to cherish and protect.
She was my heritage,
and I was her legacy. She was my past,
and I was her future.

I never saw her in this way before, but realized now, in this unlikely setting, how invaluable and precious she was to me. All honor to her.

There were three women working with my mother in her room today: one was her nurse and the other two were therapists from the physical and occupational therapy departments, who now formed the main contingent charged with the task of rehabilitating her. Generally, the two departments worked separately, as each had its own area of focus and expertise. Physical therapy emphasized more the rehabilitation of broader functions, such as sitting up, transferring, and walking, while occupational therapy highlighted specific tasks such as brushing one's teeth, writing, or dressing. As my mother required "total assistance," the two departments met together to pool their efforts and to assist each other in moving her.

My mother was an agreeable patient, they said, friendly and cooperative, but she was simply unable to do anything. With one-half of her body paralyzed, it was virtually impossible for her to execute any purposeful movement.

"Come on, Tilly," said the occupational therapist, a stout woman named Roberta who was assisting her in the task of sitting up. It was disheartening to see how so basic a movement was completely out of reach. I watched as she failed in producing even a semblance of the action. I confronted again the ever-present despair - oddly worsened since she had awaken, as if by sleeping she had better concealed the bitter reality.

"Come on, Tilly, that's it," Roberta said again, as if Mom were making any effort, which she was not. As far as I could see, Mom was doing *nothing*. She grimaced slightly, as if attempting to will the movement to occur by some sort of telepathy, but there was no discernible advance. The derelict left half now overwhelmed the functioning right – a pitiful and hopeless display. What amazed me, however, was my mother's demeanor. She seemed quite forgiving of the morass, which I found utterly surprising.

"Shift, now, Tilly. Shift. Use the right arm to balance. That's it," the therapist said enthusiastically.

Mom made some pathetic effort, simulating a kind of *virtual* movement, more imagined than actual.

I found her composure, under the circumstances, incredible, because she had never before been calm. Quite the contrary, she had always been anxious and fretted endlessly over things that were often trivial.

Roberta placed a pillow under Mom's right side to help provide some support. "Try to shift now, Tilly. Here, let me get another pillow."

I was amazed, in light of the many petty things she had agonized over, to see the serenity with which she had accepted what was in every sense a life-shattering event. It was as if the misery wrought by stroke was *so* overwhelming that she had made the utterly logical, but completely uncharacteristic decision to accept it, as if realizing that struggle against so formidable an adversary was pointless.

"Come on, Tilly, roll towards me!" commanded the youthful therapist named Sara. The briskness of her voice pierced the thick cloud of lethargy surrounding my mother. "Move your eyes this way, lead with your eyes!"

I wondered if the calm I observed in her was actually a manifestation of depression or resignation (a resignation completely at odds with the intense conflict roiling within me). But, I thought not; it seemed to run deeper than that, emanating from some other more sturdy and ennobling process within her.

"Come on, Tilly, that's it, roll this way."

She did her best but was unable to offer anything but token assistance as the therapists labored to move her to the sitting position. Their goal was to get her to sit up and transfer from side to side, to redevelop her "sitting balance," as they called it. Once they accomplished this, they could work on standing, weight shifting, pivoting, and turning. All that, though, seemed quite improbable. Having no success with sitting, they worked on simply getting her to roll over: first, to the left, her affected side, which was easier, using, as counterweight the efforts of her functioning right side. "Lead with your eyes, Tilly, and turn your head this way. Now roll over. That's it!" Sara said. There was much rooting and encouragement but little to show for it. Mom looked towards her, and that was about it. Sara placed her hand on Mom's right shoulder and clasped Mom's right hand, while Roberta nudged from behind. "Turn your head this way!" Sara said, exhorting Mom. "Then try to bring your shoulder over! Come on, we'll help you. Now your hip, rotate your hip, that's it, Mrs. Moss, keep trying!" Her words were intensely optimistic. As far as I could tell, Mom did almost *nothing*, just looking, and, perhaps, turning her head. She seemed to want to comply, but did so without effect. What was worse was that this was her good side. To roll to the right, attempting to use her affected left side would have been all but ceremonial.

"We're not having much luck, today, Tilly," Sara, said, smiling sympathetically and doing her best to avoid conveying the sense of failure she undoubtedly felt. Mom looked up at me, as if out of breath. What a thief, I thought, was stroke, preying on the innocent and the aged. I assigned evil intentions to this completely impersonal process. I forced a smile, keeping a happy face for my mother.

"Let's get her up in the chair with the Hoyer lift. We can do some range of motion," Roberta said. The nurse walked outside the room where the "Hoyer lift" was waiting. This was a motorized unit, almost like a forklift, except with a wide canvas harness instead of metal forks. They maneuvered the unit into the room and positioned the harness around her. They secured and strapped her in. Operating the control panel, as the powerful machine swung into action, they raised my mother, quite comfortably, and moved her over and down into a reclining chair next to her bed, not unlike unloading some unwieldy cargo. They removed the harness, made some minor adjustments, and amazingly Mom was sitting up. It seemed almost to transform her, as if elevating her from the utterly dependent position had similarly lifted her spirits.

The therapists began working on her left arm, hand, and fingers, flexing, extending, and rotating them, passively running them through their full range of motion.

"You generally get proximal return first," Sara said to me, meaning that the upper extremity – the hand, arm, and shoulder – began functioning before the lower extremity. The lowly foot was last in the sequence.

"What time frame are we talking about?"

"It depends, Dr. Moss. It'll take time," she said, avoiding a direct answer.

They molded Mom's left hand into a fist, then extended the fingers, placing them against the outstretched fingers of her right hand in an attitude of prayer. Then they flexed and extended the elbow. Then the shoulder.

"That's it, Tilly. Does it feel good?" the therapist asked. My mother raised her right eyebrow in affirmation. Despite the difficulty and non-existent progress, the therapists seem to like Mom, as if, even with her abbreviated modes of communication, they could detect her nuances and quirks, her sense of humor and eccentricities.

They worked on the left leg, flexing, extending, and rotating it, beginning with the hip, then the knee, and then the foot and toes. They extended Mom's toes while the therapist tapped her left knee, giving sensory reminders to her flaccid left leg.

"We have to get normal posture back before we can have movement," Sara said, looking at Mom. Mom seemed surprisingly attentive. She could do nothing with her body, but responded well to this drill sergeant of a therapist.

In Mom's case, though, there was no posture to speak of, and the movements were entirely passive. But they served their purpose, which was to stimulate her left side, prevent ulcers and contractures, reestablish normal reflexes, and, importantly, to retain the *memory* of normal body movement. I perceived a spiritual dimension to physical therapy beneath the patina of mechanical exercises and routines – a striving to recollect past lives, to recall past connections engraved into the nervous system from childhood and infancy, and before.

There were within each of us, ancient memories, almost embryologic, of migrating axons seeking out mates, synapsing with other nerves and muscle fibers by the thousands, by the millions, weaving ethereal tapestries that miraculously resulted in movement – wondrous and graceful movement that now, in retrospect, seemed almost sublime. It was the remembrance of such movement and its mechanisms, of past lives filled with activity (lives that now seemed so intolerably remote), that could rekindle the old pathways, create new ones – and heal.

"Think about the movement," the therapists urged Mom, "help me do it, bend the knee!" It was impossible, but an admonishment that pressed Mom to restore in her memory the lost image and impression of her living body and the sensation of functioning limbs. Perhaps, memory was all she had to go on – all *we* had to go on, a fractured present rendered whole somehow by the past

When the half hour session was up, the therapists returned Mom to her bed (a fate she seemed happily consigned to), packed all their utensils (including the offensive Hoyer lift), bid Mom *adieu*, and, in worker like fashion, abruptly left, having for now completed their task. I followed them out and spoke with Sara.

"Her progress is slow," she told me, "but she is doing a little better." I felt she was being polite.

"Do you think we can get her to walk again?" I asked.

"It's too early to say. She had a dense stroke."

"Do you think I can get her to stand and pivot, so she can use a bedside commode?"

"I don't want to discourage you, but you may have to consider placing her in a nursing home."

"Can we do more therapy?"

"Not really, she's having trouble with two sessions. We may have to go down to one."

I returned to Mom's room. She was worn. I was distraught.

"Come on, Ma, let's get outta here and take a walk." It was a moment of pure indulgence. Imagine the joy now of so routine a pleasure. "Y'know, we've been having such beautiful sunsets. The kind you always loved."

She looked at me, raised her right eyebrow and smiled. It was another ancient memory.

I wondered about this phenomenon of "stroke," about this wrathful deity, stroke. I wondered if there was an offering I could make to appease it, a sacrifice I could bring, wheat or corn (the best of the year's harvest), or a plump lamb or goat. I kissed my mother and offered a prayer instead. I asked my God to heal her, even as the lesser but still powerful deity, stroke, rebuffed me.

I wondered which was supreme – stroke and, by extension, nature and biology? Or faith? Or were they one and the same?

When I was very young, I identified strongly with my religion. How I came to this early attachment was through the stories my mother read to me of our past. They captivated me and possessed magic and power. They spoke of a jealous and wrathful God, who still loved his people, Israel, despite their lapses and treacheries. They told of bravery, loyalty, and of devastation. They revealed the great figures of the Old Testament, of the Hebrew Bible, who stood out like mythic heroes, men and women of valor and strength, yet human and faltering.

Each night, before bed, my mother read to me of the champions of our people. She told of Abraham, the founder of our faith, and of Noah, who built the arc. She read of Joseph, the dreamer and favorite son of Jacob, who saved the House of Israel from famine. She spoke of Moses, our greatest prophet who freed the Hebrew slaves, parted the waters, and received the Ten Commandments at Sinai. She told of David, the boy warrior-poet, who slew Goliath, and Solomon, his son, who became Israel's wisest king.

There were so many heroes, so many great men and women, all of them, my mother emphasized, part of the ancestral lineage tying us directly to God, members of our family however distant, linked by blood. With such a family, such a pantheon of ancestors to call my own, I felt my heart swirl with excitement to hear of them, swept up in visions of war and conquest, triumph and defeat, and devotion to the one true God. I loved my religion, believed fervently in its stories and myths, and absorbed myself eagerly into the faith of my fathers.

Of all the stories my mother read to me, of all the great men and women who illuminated the darkness and stirred my young soul, there was one in particular that spoke to me more deeply than the rest. That was the story of Samuel, who, as a young boy, heard the voice of God calling him.

And the Lord called Samuel again. And he arose and went to Eli, and said, here am I; for thou didst call me. And

Eli perceived that the Lord had called the child. Therefore Eli said unto Samuel, Go, lie down: and it shall be, if He calls thee, that thou shalt say, Speak, Lord; for thy servant heareth. So Samuel went and lay down in his place. And the Lord came, and stood, and called as at other times, Samuel, Samuel. Then Samuel answered, Speak; for thy servant heareth. And Samuel grew, and the Lord was with him. And all Israel knew that Samuel was established to be a prophet of the Lord.
                                                   Samuel I 3:12-20

At age six, I decided that I wanted to be a Hebrew prophet, and not just any prophet. I wanted to be Samuel.

"Ma," I said to my mother as she was preparing stuffed peppers in the kitchen, "I want to change my name."

"Uh huh."

"Did ya hear, Ma?"

"Yeah, what's that, son?"

"I'm gonna change my name."

"To what?"

"Samuel."

"Oh, yeah. Why's that?"

"I want to be a prophet."

"Oh, really? Since when?"

"I decided last night."

"How 'bout a rabbi?"

"Not a rabbi, Ma, a prophet."

"Uh huh, son, pass the salt, please."

"I heard God speak to me, Ma."

She smiled and looked at me. "Oh, really?"

"Yeah, Mom, I heard him last night. He called me and I stood up and listened and it was quiet, but I could hear a voice inside my head. He called me Samuel. I wanted to tell you but you were sleeping."

Mom kept looking at me. "Uh huh."

"I remembered the story from the Bible. And Eli told Samuel it was the voice of God."

"That's right, son."

"*And Eli told Samuel what to say to the Lord."*

"*Uh huh."*

"*And I got up in my bed and said, 'Speak, Lord, for thy servant heareth,' just like the story. I said it soft so I wouldn't wake Cliff or Jerry up, but I talked to God, Ma!"*

Mom kept staring at me. She laughed a little and said, "*OK son, Samuel."*

For the next year, I was Samuel. Mom told my teacher at school to call me Samuel, made all my brothers and friends call me Samuel, told all the aunts, uncles, and cousins to call me Samuel. She introduced me to whomever we met as Samuel. She smiled at her young prophet, saying, "*I think he wants to be a rabbi."*

"*Not a rabbi, Mom, a prophet."*

"*Oh, a prophet,"* and everyone nodded and smiled, "*yeah, a prophet. OK."* And so Mom had her little Hebrew prophet in the Bronx, helping her with the groceries and taking out the garbage.

Several months into my Samuel phase an event occurred that only intensified my belief. I awoke one morning to find a golden ring emblazoned with the Hebrew letters **shin, daled**, and **yud** resting on the stand right next to my bed.

I picked it up and held it, mystified. It seemed to radiate with brilliant amber light. It had weight and body and shimmered with godly presence. It was not there when I went to sleep. It had materialized, I believed, delivered by divine hands to my bedside as I slept.

"*Ma, what is it, how'd it get here, who brought it?"* I asked, showing her the ring. She studied it, smiling, "*I don't know, son."*

"*What is it, what do the letters say?"*

"*Shaddai, son, that's one of God's names. Put it on, Samuel, does it fit?"*

"*Yes, it does, it's beautiful."*

"*It's a gift from God, Samuel, for his little prophet."*

"*How did it get here?"*

"*I don't know, son, maybe God brought it."*

"Did any of you put it there," I asked my brothers who were eating bagels in the kitchen.

"Not me, Chubs," Jerry said. "Maybe Santa Claus put it there."

"Shut up, Mule," I answered back. "Did you get it for me, Ma," I asked.

Mom just looked at me and smiled.

Helen, Larry's girlfriend, was in the kitchen, and said, "Wear it, Samuel, just wear it, and enjoy it as a gift from God."

I never knew how it got there but accepted it as a direct transmission from the Lord, a sacred object delivered or materialized by the Almighty Himself to his young prophet. My mind and heart were more than ready to embrace such a possibility, and so I wore it as such.

In years to come, I realized it was not divine hands that had brought it, not at least directly, but those of my mother's, God's proxy in my life.

-22-

I spoke with Regan about Mom's progress. I wondered if he grew weary of my queries.

"There is not much new, Rick," he said. "It's just going to take time."

"She's always so sleepy in the morning."

"She's still recovering from the shock of the stroke."

I nodded. "You may want to start looking at nursing homes."

This comment I did not want to hear. "How much time do we have in skilled care?" I asked.

"Medicare allows you one hundred days, but she has to show continuous progress."

"A hundred days," I said pensively.

"Yeah, that's it. And that's lifetime. Not each time. Medicare gives you one hundred total lifetime days. But we'll know before then, Rick. She won't use up her allotment. She'll either make it on her own or she won't, and we'll know before then."

"Which one do you recommend?" I asked, venturing into this unknown terrain. I had no idea about how one got a patient admitted to a nursing home, how much it cost, and how the facilities stacked up against one another.

"There's Providence Home, Northwood, and Brookside."

"Right," I nodded feebly.

"Let me know if you need any help with this, Rick."

"Yeah, Bruce, thanks."

Ten days before, we were enjoying a stroll on a beautiful September night. Now we were comparing nursing homes.

As a form of meditation, I began to read about normal movement – healthy, unencumbered movement, movement undeformed, fractured, or futile: a kind of homage to robust, normal function, to vigor and strength, to wellbeing. I pulled from my shelf a book I had not looked at in years, a mighty tome that, as a medical student, I had perused for any number of eternities, a dusty old volume on Neuroanatomy, packed with particulars about nerves tracts and pathways, lemnisci and ganglia of every shade, purpose, and variation. I found bizarre solace in skimming its busy pages. I lost myself in its lines and diagrams, tables and graphs, seeing art, beauty, and grandeur everywhere somehow in its tiresome detail and tedium.

Why I should spend my time as such was not immediately apparent. The obvious explanation was that it was an attempt to paper over my wounds. The stroke that had afflicted my mother had afflicted me, as any wound to a loved one would. But I had been particularly obsessed with it, knowingly and purposely driven to confront its rude mechanism. I wanted to reach into its damp underside and rip out some vital entrail or organ and disarm it. Alas, it was not so easily undone. I did not appreciate the callous demeanor of the so-called random disease process. Inadvertently, it drove me to some impolite questions about God. It was also quite consistent with the belief system of a non-believer. Why, in a remote and impersonal universe, devoid of moral purpose, should anyone be surprised when one's mother was stricken by a stroke? Such unhappiness, it seemed, would be inevitable. Yet, despite it all, I was unwilling to abandon faith, only question it.

I felt it incumbent upon me to wonder aloud about Divine justice, as anyone experiencing tragedy may tend to. But I felt that before doing so, before questioning the Creator on the moral basis of His creation, I should reinstate balance and composure by reacquainting myself with the majesty of that creation. I would immerse myself in the study of the non-diseased state of the human organism, the perfect universe, so to speak, to inspire the proper degree of gratitude and awe before succumbing to unworthy conclusions. And, so, I studied normal movement as a balm for my wounds and as a form of religious exercise.

I visited my mother that night, almost an afterthought after an evening immersed in the yellowed pages of my Neuroanatomy text. When I arrived, I found her head slumped over as she lay in the reclining chair. A sudden wave of terror gripped me.

"Mom!" I shouted, grasping her frantically. She opened her eyes, enough to ease the pounding of my heart. She seemed to acknowledge me from some deep chasm within herself, rising to the surface just momentarily, enough for a few mumbled but precious syllables, "Hi, Rick . . ." Then a return to the depths. But it was more than just sleeping. It seemed as if she was *absent,* lost somewhere and inaccessible. I wondered if there were some obscure niche or recess where she huddled, communing with herself, gathering her energies for ordeals to come.

The NG tube continued to deliver the creamy liquid that sustained her, drop by drop. The curtain separating her from her roommate was drawn, but I could hear her roommate breathing somnolently. She was the aunt of a teacher in town who I knew, in her seventies and recovering from a hip replacement. She and my mother had become comrades, friendly faces for each other in the midst of their personal struggles. Of course, her outlook was entirely different: her hip

would heal with time and a complete recovery was expected. Not so, my mother. Perhaps, my mother's healing was of a different sort. Her profound submersions,
her unlikely calm in the midst of the tumult, all spoke
to another kind of curative. Yet, I felt this story did not
have a happy ending. She would *not* walk out of here.

A nurse entered. "Hi, Dr. Moss." Her voice grated,
or, perhaps, it was just me. "Your Mom's doing OK,"
she said in sunny fashion. "Been very tired, though.
Sleeping most of the time. I think she's worn out from
the day's therapy." She was oblivious to my fidgeting.
Just as well. I didn't need the nurses thinking that I'd
become crazed. She left the room after adjusting my
mothers tube feeding.

"Call me if you need anything."

I sat by my sleeping mother again. My routine. Now
her entire body slept, not just the left side. Stroke was
a form of sleep, an unwanted slumber for the affected
part from which there could be no arousal, or if so, only
after much time and in miserly portions. At least, while
asleep, my mother did not have to confront the permanent slumber imposed upon the left half of her body.
Stroke, then, more than sleep, was a kind of death, a
quasi-death, or worse. With death, at least, one was either joined with the Creator or without consciousness
– in either event, without suffering. But with stroke,
one could not escape the fetters of a crippled body, one
could not separate oneself from the parasitic flesh that
cleaved and foraged on the healthy side and shackled
one to a bed and a life of dependency. Was death not
better? I was no longer sure.

I wondered if there were any sparks that flew
within the frozen limbs of my mother, any glimmers or
twitches of life. Did the dormant nerve fibers that once
shuttled impulses efficiently, conveying streams of data
up and down her limbs and trunk, between body and

brain, stir even slightly now, ripple somewhere with traces of light?

She roused again. Her eyes flickered, a brief interlude of recognition, and then oblivion. Where was redemption? Jews were always looking for redemption, and if not redemption, at least reconciliation. I had not found mine. I would twist and mangle my prayers, squeeze them and extract from them my redemption. Then my studies. To liberate *myself* from the awesome grip of stroke, I would return to my studies. I would save myself through prayer and study, as the good Jew my mother raised me to be – while clasping for a reason to believe.

I returned quickly to the study of movement, my review of old chapters memorized long ago, a strange but vital haven for me. It was late, the kids were asleep, having long given up on their compulsive father, he at present gripped by phobias and no longer disposed to playing and frolicking as before. Sleep offered better options for them, and for now, this served my purposes well. I indulged myself, my obsessions, and submitted to the grim spectacle of extracting joy and sustenance from the monotonous conflations of Neuroanatomy. I continued my previous meditations on nerve and fiber, on functioning filaments and muscle.

The phenomenon of movement belied explanation; the mechanism lay hidden within the folds and fissures of our inheritance, which was to say - our anatomy. But it was not just the gross anatomy, but the subtle and hidden anatomy, the ultramicroscopic cellular anatomy of motor end plates and synapses, of vesicles and mediators, of a pyrotechnic molecular physiology, and of a dizzying complex of neural connections upon which the awesome edifice of motion was based. It was a miracle – at least, a *secular* miracle - that a finger, foot, or face, could move with such precision and skill, exactly when we wanted and how.

We spoke, kissed, wrote, and walked without pause, never considering the sorcery, the wizardry, the overwhelming intelligence behind it. But how did such ballet occur, with the mere thought, and if all things wished for as extraordinary as this could be willed into existence so easily! It was a miracle that one could grasp a pencil, write a letter, sit up in a chair, stand and pivot, walk, run, or ride a bicycle! And if one were casual about such commonalities, then contemplate the body unable to perform, the body magnificent stricken by *stroke:* the paralysis, the frozen sinew, the numbness, and contractures. Where once there was untrammeled movement, unfettered composition, there was now only deep anesthesia, whole portions of bodies ruined (and, thusly, lives), condemned to a netherworld and unhappy irony: warm to touch and pink in color yet crippled and devoid of vigor.

Commonplace movement was worthy of reflection. I pondered its mystery and witchcraft, no, the engineering brilliance behind the *miracle* of movement. I probed and explored this vast and once familiar terrain. And for my mother, she, at least, had one half of her body that she could willfully summon. In good conscience, I could consider this brief incursion a celebration of that which was still alive and well with her, a tribute to her functioning right side – and to the grandeur of creation. Perhaps, faith was still possible.

I paused momentarily from my studies, folding the page and closing the book. It was beautifully illustrated, the color renditions easily tracked, making the amazing confluence of pathways comprehensible. I looked at the clock, its ticking somehow soothing, and saw that it was almost midnight. I scanned the items on my desk, a collection of pieces from around the world. My eyes settled on one such item: an arabesque from Spain. It was inlaid with fragments of wood, jade, and alabaster, of repeating geometric patterns, with lines of inlaid gold leaf dividing it into exquisite sections. I took a deep breath, half wondering why I was up so late and the reasons for my preoccupations. My mother had a stroke; she was 78. These things happened, of course. I knew that.

And I knew that I digressed. My whole life had been a series of digressions. Going into medicine was a digression. Leaving the country for several years was a digression. But this digression into study was different. I did it in order to breathe.

I looked over once more the tracts and ganglia and synapses involved in lifting one's pinkie and shuddered at the complexity. Movement, precise, controlled, and exquisite movement, sometimes simple, sometimes elaborate, *was* extraordinary. What was extraordinary about it was the flawlessness and ease with which it was performed – a flawlessness based on the all-consuming genius that founded it. But because the grace, precision, and informality of movement all teetered at the summit of this astonishingly complex and integrated system, this dense forest of fibers, tracts, and nerves, the entire venture was poised to stumble with the slightest breach.

Was it any wonder that a stroke affecting a relatively small portion of the central nervous system, but in a critical area, such as the internal capsule, could throw the whole enterprise into disarray – the sprawling apparatus completely undone by a peanut sized disruption? As interwoven and tightly connected as the system was, a well-placed cerebral infarct easily affected the affairs of a multitude of distant effector (motor) neurons in the spinal cord and elsewhere. With motor neurons thusly abandoned, bereft of proper guidance from oracles above (the cerebral cortex), they, of necessity, forsook their once active and obedient confederates, the muscles, to a destiny of flaccidity and atrophy, and then later, of rigidity and spasm, transformed into

a knot of contorted bands where once there was gliding, lustrous sinew. And with muscles thusly censured,
movement, of course, ceased.

Such was the extraordinary circuitry behind the
simple task of lifting one's pinkie (or any other movement), the marvel of motion, of purposeful activity, and
the despair behind the vascular event known as stroke.

When I closed the book for the last time that night, I
felt relieved. I reflected. It seemed restful to do so. Then
other memories dawned and took hold, dim recollec-
tions long forgotten, of the pain and suffering she had
endured . . .

*It was a few months after the circus when I next saw
my father. He no longer visited. It was too painful for everyone. I loved my father. He was good to us, played with
us in a way that only fathers could – picking us up, calling
us "little monkeys," taking us for rides in his car, throwing
firecrackers out the window, raising hell in general. But his
visits demoralized my mother for weeks. I was not glad that
he stopped visiting, but I knew it was better that he did .*

*There was peace in the house, an agitated peace, if one
can call it such, with a nervous, brooding mother watching
over her family, doing our laundry, cooking meals, and earn-
ing a meager salary as a secretary.*

*When I returned from school one day, Jerry told me he
had seen Dad. Jerry was ten and I was seven.*

"Where?" I asked excitedly.

"At the Crossroads on Boston Road."

"What's that?"

"A bar."

"What's a bar?" I asked.

"Where people drink."

"Drink what?"

"Liquor. Never mind. Different things."

"How did he get there?"

"By train."

"Is he with anyone?"

"Other people. They sit there, talk, drink, and eat peanuts. Ya wanna go?" Jerry asked.

"What for?"

"Whaddaya mean 'what for?' To see Dad!"

"What about Mom?"

"He's your Dad."

"Should we ask Mom?"

"No!"

"Whaddaya say to him?"

"Nothin'. I don't let him see me."

After supper, I told Mom I was going to the playground with Jerry. We went down Crotona Park East to Boston Road.

We walked past the Associated, the cleaners where Linda got shot, Tony's Pizza place, the Dover movie theater, the candy store, and came to a dark little place with a sign over the entrance that said "Crossroads." There were neon signs on the windows and two large wooden doors. I looked at Jerry.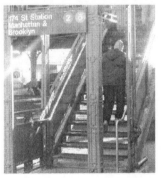

"Can we go in?"

"Wait for Dad."

"I don't wanna wait for Dad. Ya mean he's not in there?"

"Not yet, he usually gets here in a few minutes, around seven." There was a big clock hanging in the window. "It's five to seven," Jerry said.

We waited behind a car. "I don't like this," I said.

"It's OK."

"Ya think Dad will mind?"

"Naa, it'll be fine."

A few minutes later, we heard the train roll in at the 174th Street station. Then we saw the familiar silhouette of my father walking down the stairs from the "El," to the land-

ing, and into the street. It was dark already, so he couldn't see us. He was wearing the long grey coat he always liked, smoking a cigarette, taking a big drag as he walked past us. I got so excited I almost yelled out, but Jerry grabbed me and put his finger to his lips. "Shhh," he said quietly. I heard Dad's familiar cough as he opened the doors of the bar to walk in.

"Wait a few minutes," Jerry said.

"Why? I wanna see Dad."

"Just shut up and wait a minute."

A few minutes passed. Jerry looked both ways and said, "Let's go." He went first, and I followed him into the bar. There was a second door. Then we were inside. It was dark with music on and a fog of cigarette smoke hanging in the air. There were tables and chairs, a jukebox, a long wooden counter, and stools where men sat in hats and overcoats, hunched over glasses, smoking and drinking. There were two bartenders behind the counter. Behind them were mirrors and rows of bottles lined up against the wall. No one noticed us. I tried to find Dad.

"Come here," Jerry said, pulling me over to a table in the corner next to the outside window where no one could see us. Then I saw Dad walk out of the bathroom. I almost yelled his name, but Jerry grabbed me.

"Why can't I talk to Dad?"

"Not now."

"Why not?"

"Because this is a bar!"

"So what?"

"You drink here."

"Drink what?"

"Liquor."

"What's that?"

"Alcohol."

"What Mom rubs on us when we have a fever?"

"No you idiot! Whiskey. And we're not supposed to be here!"

Dad sat down at the counter. He took a drag on his ciga-
rette and had a drink. He coughed a little. He flicked his ciga-
rette into the ashtray. I wanted to say something, but Jerry
squeezed my arm. We sat for a few minutes, watching my
father smoke and drink. A few minutes later, a blonde-haired
woman walked in wearing a shiny necklace, high heels, and
cherry lipstick. She hung up her coat and walked over to
where Dad was sitting. Dad smiled, said something, as if
he knew her. She sat down and gave Dad a kiss. She held his
hand and ordered a drink.

"Who's that?" I asked.

"I don't know. She comes here to meet him."

"Why's Dad kissing her?"

"I guess he likes her, stupid."

"What about Mom?"

"Mom and Dad don't get along."

"But he shouldn't be kissing her."

"You don't know anything, Rick."

"It's not fair," I said. Jerry rolled his eyes.

"I'm going to see Dad." I got up. Jerry grabbed me.

"You little jerk!" he yelled.

"You're the jerk!" I said, and we began scuffling. I pushed
him and walked toward Dad. Jerry grabbed me from behind.
I tried to squirm away. He wrestled me to the floor, knocking
over a chair. A few people turned. Then Dad turned. I saw his
face. Jerry let me go. I stood up.

"Hi, Dad," I said smiling. He looked at me, cigarette
dangling from his mouth, the smoke rising in little circles
around his dark hair. He coughed. He took a drag from his
cigarette. He didn't smile. I was surprised that he didn't
seem happy to see me. The lady moved her hand away from
Dad. She looked at Dad, then at me. She smiled. I looked at
her and then at Dad.

"Hello," she said. I smiled. "Is this one of your kids,
Harry?" I nodded, but Dad didn't say anything. Then Jerry
walked over, and the two of us stood before Dad in the middle
of the bar.

"Hi, Dad," Jerry said weakly.

Dad looked at him, dragging on his cigarette and blowing smoke through his nose. He coughed. He moved his eyes back and forth between his two sons.

"Whaddaya doin' heah," he said finally, his voice low and menacing, looking at Jerry, the older one.

"Uhh, nothing, Dad."

"Uh huh," Dad said, still looking at Jerry. "You always stop by bars, kid?"

"N-no, just once in a while."

"I see. Whudaboutchoo?" he said to me.

"Not me Dad, this is my first time. But Jerry told me you always came here."

Dad stared at Jerry.

"You spyin' on ya old man?" Dad asked.

"Nooo," Jerry said, shaking his head stupidly.

"You shouldn't be takin' ya kid brudda heah either."

The lady stood up, as if to leave.

"Who are you," I asked.

"Uh, I-I'm – a friend of your father's."

"What's your name?" I asked.

"Uh, well–"

"Never mind, kid," Dad said.

"How long have you known my Dad?"

She smiled awkwardly. "Well - uh - not long." She looked at Dad.

"She's just a friend, kid."

I wanted to ask her how long she'd been kissing my dad when Dad stood up. He reached into his pocket and pulled out a couple of quarters.

"Heah ya go, kids. Now donlemme catch ya heah again."

"Thanks, Dad," we said. Jerry and I walked toward the door. I took a few steps and turned.

"When ya coming home, Dad?" I asked. Dad looked at me.

"I dunno little monkey," he said, and for the first time he smiled. "Ya mudda an' I don' get along too well."

I wanted to cry when I heard this.

"Kid?"

"Yeah, Dad."

"Don't tell ya mudda ya saw me today, heah?"

We walked home. We were quiet for a while and then I asked, "Whose Dad's friend?"

"Shuddup, Ricky."

"Why don't you shut up? You're the one who brought me there."

When we got home it was already late for a school night, and Mom was angry. She asked me where we went. "To a bar," I said.

Jerry immediately began contorting his face.

"Whaddaya mean a bar?" Mom asked.

"'The Crossroads Bar.'" Jerry twisted his face some more.

"We saw Dad there," I said. Jerry held his neck as if he were choking. Mom stared at me.

"What was he doing there?"

"He was drinking."

"With who?"

"A friend."

Mom's eyes narrowed. "Who was this 'friend'?" Jerry's face now screwed up into a little red ball.

"Some lady. She had blonde hair and wore cherry lipstick. She had a sparkly necklace."

Mom looked at me. Jerry kept shaking his head, his eyes about to burst.

"And she kissed Dad."

Mom almost gasped when she heard this. Her face grew pale. Tears began to form. "Bastard," she said as she looked at us angrily. "Don't go near him again! Do you hear me? Never again!" She ran into the kitchen.

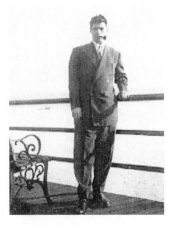

"*Stupid idiot!*" *Jerry said, swatting me in the back of the head.*

I heard Mom crying. I went to see her. She was sitting on a chair, holding her head over the table. I put my arm around her. She looked at me. She stroked my face. She smiled even as the tears rolled down her cheeks. Then she got me a glass of milk. She asked if I had done my homework. She walked me to my bed and tucked me in. She kissed me goodnight. Then she went back to the kitchen. Jerry yelled at me for ratting on Dad. I felt unhappy and full of guilt. I heard Mom crying as I drifted off to sleep.

- 23 -

I visited my mother after hours, as was my custom, and found her sitting up in a reclining chair, placed there by the nurses with the help of the Hoyer lift. I had been seeing her twice daily, sometimes even three times, but she was usually sleeping. So I came mostly in the evenings when she was more alert.

These visits to my ailing mother were of a genre of experience that most people eventually went through in their lives, and something in it seemed proper and natural, a necessary phase that brought order to life, however unhappy. In executing such tasks, one assured that one paid fitting attention to the elderly and infirm of one's family, those who had suffered and labored on one's behalf through the decades, as the younger themselves were now consumed by struggle.

As I walked over from my office, I felt as if I were putting on a uniform and assuming a role – that of dutiful son. Yet I took solace in it, wore the colors proudly, as if the drive or moral impetus to perform this were welded into me, the cryptic directives buried deep within those very same ganglia and nerve tracts that I had been preoccupied with of late. It was as much a function of biology as socialization, part of our innate temperament, so to speak, as if nature had designed us to perform such tasks to allow for the necessary transition of the generations. Life, at its most atomized, pivoted on this small and simple arrangement between

family members, in keeping with fundamental principles, as akin to the natural order as the passage of the
seasons.

As I entered her room, I had a particular worry
quite apart from the usual concerns. She had always
been open in her devotions, but the deeper areas of her
life remained hidden, screened off by walls, to which
stroke only added another layer. Yet, when I saw her
this time, she appeared more animated, more alert than
anytime since the event, now twelve days ago.

"Hi, Ricchh," she said, raising her right eyebrow,
her speech still slurred.

"How are ya, Mom?" I asked drearily. I kissed her
and held her paralyzed left hand. It was odd, but there
was a role reversal here. I was in good health, yet despondent, while my invalid mother cheered me.

"Fine, Rick," she said. "How are you?" She sounded bubbly. How could it be?

My mother's affect concerned me, although that
may seem curious. I had been trying to discern whether
her calm demeanor reflected some inexplicable change
in her emotional make-up, or the surface patina of depression. She had developed through the years mechanisms of denial, and, presumably, they were still in
effect. But this seemed different. There was missing in
her persona the usual tics and twitches that exposed
the lie. She seemed truly to hover above the morass,
somehow removed from the wrenching disruption of
her illness.

"How do you feel, Mom?"

Her right eyebrow shot up, she shrugged and said
OK, and truly she did not seem perturbed.

"Are you OK with all this?" I probed again.

She had built her walls before out of necessity, but
no such urgency existed now.

Her eyebrow went up again. "I'm OK, Rick," she
said, and she smiled beautifully.

I was disarmed. Was she telling the truth? She had always been skillful at evasion, at looking at her agony obliquely, as if playing a role. But I knew she relived the painful images over and over, dissecting her memories completely, yet disclosing nothing. And she refused to let them go. We could never touch them, the inner frailties; never inquire into how she actually felt; nor would she ever tell. But there was something different now, not pathologic at all, in fact, quite the opposite. My confusion arose because it collided with the experience of the last forty years. Had she undergone some internal restructuring, drank from some pool of liberating insight that enabled her to adapt herself and transform life-altering events into trifles to be conformed to with ease?

"So you're really OK with this, Ma? Stuck in the hospital, can't move or get up? It's OK?"

"Rick," she said with an air of indifference, "what's the use of complaining?"

She smiled as if amused. I felt as if I was with a stranger. But I could live with this alter ego of my mother. "If there's something on your mind, Ma," I said, "please tell me."

Was the old religion at work? She had dedicated herself to it and passed it on dutifully to her children. Was she now enjoying the fruits of her devotion? Had God taken the initiative, healing her inwardly even as her body lay broken? It all seemed uncanny to me, so unexpected. But, if my mother was without anguish or torment in the aftermath of a major stroke, then how could I complain?

"The speech therapist told me your swallowing has improved." She looked at me as if to say, Big deal. "They want to start feeding you."

She shrugged.

Were there other mundane reasons for her unlikely calm? I wondered if being away from her phone and mailbox had something to do with it, away from the incessant calls from sons and relatives, away from the clamor and untidiness of her life.

Until the stroke, my mother had been susceptible to any imperfection in the weave of the day; a simple phone call could set her off. How many times had I heard her agonize over her sons or grandsons, Uncle Willy, Israel, the Jewish people in general, or a disaster in some far-flung corner of the world? She was vulnerable to any plea for help, a relative having a rough go of it, a synagogue in need of funds, an earthquake in Central America, what have you. But, mostly it was the family that threw her into a spell.

"Call Jack, Rick, he needs a boost," she would tell me. Or, "Did you give your Uncle Willy a call, he's not doing well." Or, "Did you speak with Harold (her grandson)? He's down in the dumps." As she aged, she became less resistant to this sort of thing, less able to absorb the punishment of bad news or even the low-grade attrition of chronic woes. She identified with those relatives in greatest distress and lacked mechanisms to defend herself against the emotional assaults.

From the mail, she received a barrage of reports on famine, bloodshed, and natural disasters from a multitude of relief organizations, all of which touched her deeply. She managed to get herself on the mailing list for nearly every charity or Jewish advocacy group and could not resist the unending accounts of hardship and requests for aid. But there was only so much that an aging lady of limited means could do.

She also received her weekly copies of the *Jewish Week* and other such Jewish periodicals, including stories on anti-Semitism and hostility towards Israel, all worthy and proper subjects for a Jewish newspaper, but quite upsetting to her.

"Don't read it, Mom, it's gonna drive you crazy," I would tell her.

"I can't stand it, Rick. They just don't give Israel a break."

"It's been going on for fifty years, Mom, there's nothing you can do."

"I can't stand that lousy Arafat!"

"He's a thief and a scoundrel," I said.

"I don't trust him."

"He's a thug."

"He should only croak," she said.

"May he drop dead as we speak," I said.

"I pray, Rick, that Israel should live in peace."

"Someday," I said.

Unable to help herself, the only way out of the torment was to remove her from the source, away from the twin engines of her anguish, the phone and the mail. Here in Indiana she could escape. But there was more to it than that. Something, indeed, was different. As I watched her relaxing, somehow at ease with all that had happened, I reflected again on her embattled past, her days of uncertainty and contention when her reactions had not been so sanguine.

Shortly after the bar incident, there began a period when my mother cried every day. It went on for months. With each episode, I felt a deep sense of helplessness. I would hold her hand and try to console her. She would look down at me through moist eyes, caressing my face. I was unable to fathom such behavior. I knew of pain and even of death and of my father. But I was also pudgy, round, and cheerful, and the world to me was still a sunny place. I loved my brothers and my mother, my aunts, uncles, and cousins, my friends and my baseball mitt and the New York Yankees and my neighborhood, playground, and school. There seemed nothing wrong with all this, and I wished only that her tears would cease, so that I could bask in the pleasure of my little world.

One brisk fall day, my mother and I were walking through Crotona Park. The day was beautiful, with rich autumn colors, yet I sensed unhappiness. I felt it in the tightness of her grip and the quickness of her gait. She was distracted and her face tense, her eyes lost in a sea of turbulent thought. A new cycle of tears seemed imminent.

I listened to the familiar sounds, the low-pitched glottal stops, the snorts and whimpering that quickened and gathered strength, her agitated breathing as she drew air through her nose in rapid jerks, her chest convulsing. Yet, despite this, she continued walking, as if it were all quite ordinary – strolling with her son and weeping hysterically. She did not reach for a tissue, cover her face, or in any way attempt to conceal it. She carried on in this manner, active and purposeful, maintaining her stride, as if by the vigor of her gait she could preserve some semblance of mental balance.

Something strange then occurred. My mother stopped and looked at me. And she asked me a question I would never forget, because she had never mentioned him before, nor would she ever again.

"Rick," she asked, almost surreptitiously, as if divulging some sinister secret. "Do you miss your father?" The question seemed to torment her, as if arising from some pool of wretchedness within her.

"Yes," I replied.

The simple response seemed to jolt her; she was bewildered but only briefly. She blinked her eyes and nodded weakly. Then, just as suddenly, she turned away, and we continued our walk.

She never mentioned him to me again, nor could I bring it up to her. She would not allow us to see him, nor him us, nor would she ever disclose her feelings about him. She would never allow the bitterness to diminish, the emotional hold he had over her to lessen, even decades later as she lie convalescing.

- 24 -

I had arranged to meet with Rabbi Goldstein, a man in his fifties, whom I had met years ago. I sought him out as I remembered him as a religious and learned man who was very serious about his faith.

"I see the study of stroke as an extension of prayer," I said.

He nodded agreement.

"But how so?" I inquired.

"Because it can be an act of devotion and God hears you when you call upon him."

"Why else?" I said, looking for a line of logic beyond simple faith – or, perhaps, the logic of healing based on faith.

"The study of Torah," he began, warming to the topic, "is equal to the study of all things. Therefore, serious study of any worthy subject and certainly the study of medicine would qualify, would be an extension of Torah study. In the preliminary prayers of the morning service, we thank God for the proper functioning of the body, without which we would be unable to stand before Him. 'Blessed are you, HaShem, Who heals all flesh and acts wondrously.' We can extrapolate from this that it would be good to study medicine." ("HaShem" means "the name." It is another name for God.)

"Where is that?" I asked, thumbing through my Siddur (Hebrew prayer book).

"Page fifteen."

"'. . . Source of our health and strength; we give You thanks and praise . . .'" I read aloud.

"Yes, that's it."

"Good. Is there anything else?" I asked.

"The '*Amidah.*' The petitionary prayer for healing," he said.

I flipped through the prayer book.

"'. . . Heal us, O, Lord, and we shall be healed, save us, O, God, and we shall be saved . . .'"

"It is said that angels or human beings can be agents of God for healing, but that such healing may be temporary or incomplete. When God Himself acts to cure someone, it will be complete, a perfect healing," he added.

"Can healing occur on a spiritual or emotional level, even if the body remains broken?"

"That, too, would be a blessing."

"And death?" I asked. "Can death be a form of healing?"

"There is a proper time for death, perhaps, the ultimate healing, when we are put to rest under the shelter of His wing."

"What else, Rabbi?"

"The '*Mi Shebeirach,*' the prayer for a sick person."

"Can we ask for grace?"

"Yes, we can ask for God's grace."

"And *Shekinah?* The Christians speak of the 'holy spirit.' Do we believe in such a thing? Can we ask for God's holy spirit?"

He furrowed his brow. "We would use another word. 'Holy Presence' might be better, so as not to confuse things." He smiled and played with his beard.

"What about neuropeptides?" He flipped an eyebrow. "I've been reading from the alternative medicine literature about the relationship between emotions and the immune system, how prayer or meditation can have a salutary effect on immune function," I said.

"When science supports the act of prayer, it is a blessing," he responded without batting an eye. He seemed quite comfortable in the realm of faith – surprising, I felt, for a modern American Jew, even if a rabbi.

"What about guilt?"

"There is a prayer for forgiveness."

"May I appeal directly to Him?"

"Yes, of course."

"When did Jews start praying?" I asked.

"There has been prayer since the Biblical period. It was formalized in the time of Ezra and Nehemiah, after the return from the Babylonian exile. It became even more important with the destruction of the Second Temple."

"The Rabbinic period?"

"Yes."

"Is there a scriptural basis to prayer as well?"

"Yes, there is."

"Do you believe in the power of prayer?" I asked.

"Yes, of course. What would I be if I didn't?"

"Even with a medical background, I can believe?" I asked, if only to hear his affirmation.

"Everyone can have faith."

He had helped me. Prayer and study were reflections of one another, as were faith and reason.

Perhaps through both prayer and study, I could better engage God to aid my mother. And so I would continue to do both.

When I walked off the elevator onto the skilled care unit, the nurses directed me to the patient lounge. There, I saw my mother sitting up in her reclining chair, NG tube and IV still in, wearing a bib. Rebecca, the speech therapist, was helping Mom with lunch.

"Hi, Mom, you look good," I said. She smiled and did not give me an annoyed "don't patronize me look" for which I was grateful. She, in fact, did appear more energetic than usual.

There was a tray in front of her with a selection of soft foods: custard, jello, pureed meat, and mashed potatoes.

"She's doing well for her first day eating, Dr. Moss," Rebecca said as she lifted another spoonful of custard to her mouth.

I watched Mom receive the custard, move it slowly to the back of her throat, and swallow.

"Keep the chin down, Tilly (my mother's preferred name). Now swallow a few times," she said.

She watched my mother complete the elementary tasks and then asked, "How are you?"

"Ok," Mom answered.

"Good." Rebecca glanced at me: "Her voice is clear and she didn't cough. That means she's not aspirating."

I smiled at Mom, who gave me a sarcastic sort of shrug and roll of her eyes.

A week before, when she had last tried eating, part of the food came pouring out of the paralyzed left side of her mouth, and the rest she aspirated, leaving her choking and sputtering. Now, she was handling custard - a sign of progress, however limited. How odd, I thought, that I should find reason for hope at the sight of my mother wearing a bib.

Rebecca turned Mom's head to the left, her weak side, and then tilted her head to the right. "This will direct the food to her strong side," she said. "Now, chin down, Tilly."

She placed another teaspoon of custard into my mother's mouth. I noticed that she placed it deliberately on the right side. "Her strong side," Rebecca said.

I watched Mom struggle with this latest food challenge. Upon completing it, Rebecca again told her to swallow several times. "Now clear the throat."

She obeyed, albeit weakly. "Now, cough, Tilly, clear the residue." She coughed. "Now swallow again."

Mom complied.

"How are you now, Tilly?"

"Fine," she said in a strong voice.

"Her voice is clear," Rebecca said, almost triumphantly.

I wondered if my mother could hold herself above the degradations.

Rebecca had taken out a small heated dental mirror. She showed the small object to my mother. She touched it to her lips, then to the tip of her tongue. Then, she began stroking the left side of my mother's tongue. She asked Mom to swallow several times. And, indeed, after the *thermal stimulation,* as she called it, her swallowing proceeded at a faster clip. "Better, Tilly," she said.

My mother seemed oblivious to all this. She was wearing her bathrobe, her grey hair combed, without make up, sitting upright in her reclining chair. She complied with the bizarre instructions and humiliations, but appeared impassive. Her eyes were attentive, yet distant, monitoring, perhaps, those recalcitrant mood rhythms that had always plagued her.

"Now, I'll stimulate the gag reflex, OK?" My mother nodded. I watched as she lowered the mirror from the tonsil to the base of the tongue and, lo, a swallow ensued, an invocation of the primitive gag reflex, missing since the devastation, but now happily returning to take its place in the orchestra of the body.

"Weak, but present," Rebecca said.

It was an odd circuit for my embattled mother, I thought, as I felt the sun stream in through the open windows. She had always managed to maneuver on the periphery of her frailties, willing them aside as was required by the urgencies of her life, but how to reconcile this? Could she find pleasure in just being alive, sensate, aware of herself and others, capable of communicating, but unable really to *do* anything?

Rebecca then took a gauze pad, dipped it into a cup of apple juice and placed it into my mother's mouth. She positioned it on the center of Mom's tongue, and said, "Push the gauze over to the right side and chew on it." This my mother accomplished readily. When Rebecca asked her to move it to the left side, she could not. She forced Mom through a tongue exercise routine, making Mom move her tongue left, right, up, down, forward, back, and then against the resistance of a wooden tongue blade. Then Mom repeated several times the consonants /t/, /d/, and /g/, and the sentence "she should show me the shirt."

The battle with her mutinous tongue continued. Mom began a series of oral movements including sticking her tongue out, pulling it back, moving it around in a circle, one way then another, opening and closing the mouth, puckering the lips as in a kiss, moving the tongue as if licking a popsicle, smiling and saying 'eee,' repeating certain sound combinations rapidly such as 'ma-ma-ma' or 'ka-ka-ka.'

Mom performed dutifully but stoically.

At last, Rebecca returned to the custard. After this grand tour of oral drill, it now seemed a welcome reprieve. My mother maintained her air of benign resignation. It was not just fatigue or neglect; rather, it was some internal accounting process, as if tabulating the seconds before the annoyances would cease.

Rebecca placed a spoonful of custard into my mother's mouth, coached her, and watched her slowly maneuver it to the back of the throat. The swallow reflex then took over, lackadaisical but effective; the weak pharyngeal contractions followed, squeezing the bolus of custard past the larynx, past the upper esopha-

geal sphincter, and into the esophagus, where it successfully wound its way down to her stomach. Rebecca
had her repeat this, staying with her, forcing her attention back to this reality, the reality of her stroke, and the
horrendous incompetence of her body.

"Wonderful, Tilly."

"Good, Mom," I added.

Her right eyebrow went up: the big deal look.

Rebecca wiped her face and removed the bib. "I'll
be in tomorrow." She smiled as she left.

If her new master, stroke, was cruel, Mom did not
seem to mind, only relieved to be done with the absur-
dities. The warm sunlight filtering into the room now
preoccupied her.

"Is it warm out, Rick?"

"Yeah, Mom." She nodded and smiled.

"You did well." She looked at me as if controlling
an urge to laugh.

"Sure," was all she said.

I kissed her goodbye and left her basking in the
sunlight that she had always loved. She did not appear
unhappy.

*When we were young, living together in the Bronx, I
remember kissing the mezuzah, the small metal box affixed to
the doorpost of our apartment. Within it lay the small parchment containing the "Shema," Judaism's most sacred prayer.
My mother taught me this, she, who never failed to kiss the
mezuzah upon entering or leaving the home.*

*"Kiss the mezuzah," she would say after kissing it her-
self, and obediently I would comply, raising my hand up towards the small, smooth metal case with the Hebrew letter,
"shin" written on it for* **Shaddai,** *the Almighty. I touched it
and then brought my fingers to my lips. If any of the brothers
were there, they would also kiss it. None of us knew what the
mezuzah was, or what it contained, beyond some vague sense*

that it was something "Jewish." Perhaps, even my mother did not know what it meant or how it came to be that Jewish homes affixed mezuzahs on their doorposts. But the tradition was there; she had learned it as a child and passed it on faithfully to us.

On special occasions like a wedding or Bar Mitzvah, kissing the mezuzah was particularly important: "Kiss the mezuzah," she would say forcefully, in case any of us thought we could slip by without observing this necessary rite. "Kiss the mezuzah," she repeated when one son had finished and the next one moved up until all five had filed past. When we were younger, Mom or one of the older brothers would pick up the smaller ones to kiss the mezuzah. If we were rushing out the door with our baseball bats and gloves, we stopped briefly to kiss the mezuzah before running down the stairs. If we were carrying shopping bags full of groceries into the house, we put them down to kiss the mezuzah. Whatever our personal thoughts about it may have been or the inconveniences of the moment, Mom had successfully drilled the importance of this small act into our minds, and, in her presence at least, we never failed to kiss the mezuzah.

I felt peculiar kissing the metal object, especially around non-Jewish friends, but generally conformed, hearing her voice somewhere in the back of my mind. "Kiss the mezuzah," I heard the voice say and obeyed.

The **Shema***, I learned later, was the founding principle of the Jewish faith that spoke of the unity of God. It was recited at least twice a day, in the morning and evening prayer services (and also upon awakening and before going to sleep), part of the revelation given to Moses and spoken by him more than three millennia ago:*

"Hear, O, Israel, the Lord is our God, the Lord is one."
(Deuteronomy 6:4-9)

The mezuzah, the metal or wooden box housing the parchment upon which were written these words was itself *sacred, the holy vault within which lay the words of the **Shema**. To touch the tiny, metal box was to bind with that which was sublime and transcendent; to merge, however briefly, with the great chain of tradition and spirituality that joined the generations of our people stretching back in time through epochs and foreign lands. It hearkened back to that eternal moment when God interceded in human history and chose the children of Israel as the vehicle with which to deliver His word (His Torah).*

The little box was a consecrated nucleus of spirituality; it had gravity and emitted force. You reached up to touch it, your fingers alighting on it, almost caressing it, as if it were something living. You brought your fingers to your lips and a synapse occurred, connecting God's word to your lips, and, hence, to your heart. Every time you entered and exited your home, it reminded you of who you were and what you came from.

As a Jew, you were part of a lineage and people that dated back to the revelation of God's Law at Mount Sinai. It said that the word of God (and God himself through His word) was near. It told vis-itors that this was a Jewish home, a sanc-tuary, an extension of the original tem-ple of Solomon, the family living here absorbed and bound by the ancient He-brew faith. The mezuzah was the first sign that the God of Israel lived within these walls.

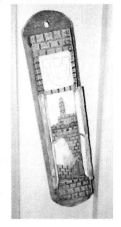

I remembered this whenever I kissed the mezuzah upon entering my own home, even as I remembered my mother who had accorded me this sacrament.

- 25 -

I scanned the article, enjoying some of the principles laid out in the opening paragraphs. It began with general comments about the unhappy fact that despite the volumes of research and trials done to prevent or reduce ischemic damage in stroke patients that a fair number of them, despite all measures, developed permanent damage. Failure of acute phase treatment (before the infarct had established itself), however, did not rule out other methods of improving recovery.

The worthy search for agents that reduced ischemic damage was inevitably limited by the short window of time one had before permanent damage occurred. Hence, only a small number of patients benefited. It was necessary, therefore, to recognize the vastly greater numbers that could profit by producing effective counterattacks once the damage had already occurred. This, briefly, was the philosophical bend of the piece. It seemed, more and more, the articles I reviewed expressed such sentiments. None of this, of course, would benefit my mother.

I looked over at the clock. It was late. I had been reading for several hours. Articles, chapters in textbooks, material taken from the Internet. When I returned home from the office, I ate supper by myself and then immediately retreated to my study in the basement where my kids would not find me. I was not interested in playing with them or even talking with my wife. I had completely altered my routines and allowed the process to overtake me, assuming new solitary patterns like a monk in a monastery. For what? I still did not know. To reconcile faith and science? The source of my duress was vague to me. I realized I was obsessed, yet did nothing to mollify it. I knew what I wanted but entertained no illusions of realizing that goal. In the meantime, I had allowed the structure and form of my life to unravel. My mother was lying in bed, paralyzed, with scant likelihood of improving, and I desperately sought to alter that brutal reality. I wanted to cure her. Whether I could succeed did not seem to matter. It consumed me, and that was all. I had reasons for my mania. That I was irrational was obvious. My center of gravity was tilting. Study consoled me. I picked up the article and read it again, this, and all the other research materials, my new compass. I was on a hunt, driven to pacify some hunger within me.

I recalled the uselessness of previous gambits into the world of stroke literature. I remembered my conversation with the Rabbi, seeing this as an extension of prayer, the two efforts somehow linked. Yet, I knew I would find nothing. I had a sense of futility, of scratching away at layers of dirt and grit, attempting to uncover an object of value, only to find it had already crumbled and disintegrated.

The hour was late. Night sounds surrounded me. Everyone was asleep in the house. I fingered the pages, underlining key phrases like a neurotic, looking for sustenance in words. How could I expect to unearth a remedy that would deliver us, my mother and me; what vanities compelled me? I could protect her no more than I could stop a determined thief or murderer. I began to see stroke in such terms, murderous and resolute. Only I was attempting to stalk *it*, looking for resolution where none could be found.

The Rabbi had elevated my worthless efforts to the level of holiness, equal to that of prayer or even the study of Torah. He had extrapolated neatly the basis for such a conclusion with the preponderance of three thousand years of tradition supporting it. One could even see the earnest study of *knitting* as holy. All were extensions of Torah study. Torah was the equal of all things. God endowed us with the ability to think and learn. Study was a holy act, in accordance with the principal of *stewardship,* with my mother's well being at stake. To accept such a notion was no different than accepting the efficacy of prayer.

Why should it be that uttering certain formulae each day invested one with any measure of holiness? It was a question of faith. So, by extension, was study. It served as a form of worship. These tortured efforts at studying, so obviously futile in materially aiding my mother, I could at least see as expressions of praise and honor to Him.

I looked at the clock, listening to its ticking. I stared at the four corners that surrounded me, the almond colored walls, the stenciled pink and purple flowers, frivolous and decorative patterns, folding lazily. Over my desk hung a painting from Nepal, an image of Tara, one of the Buddhist Bodhisattvas revered by Tibetans. It had a black background, highlighted by fiery oranges and reds, bordered by flames and lotuses, deities and demons, absorbed in their meditations, burning in their designs: a gift from a patient during the time I spent working in Katmandu as visiting surgeon. On the other wall hung a series of carved masks and pottery from Mexico and Guatemala.

I enclosed myself in my four corners, locked in my little world, looking for something redemptive. The article suggested that rehabilitation helped, that intensive therapy produced faster and more complete recovery. Other studies confirmed their findings. Self-care was more important than gross activity such as ambulation. Activities like eating, washing, and brushing ones teeth took precedence over getting up and walking.

There was more about amphetamines and other agents such as Dopamine that seemed to enhance recovery. Various mechanisms were suggested, none with certainty. The important thing was that they were looking for methods of pharmaceutical intervention *after* stroke had occurred.

But there was nothing available now – unless you were a rat or guinea pig. Then there was rehab. And the ADLs (activities of daily living). At least it had dawned on them to look in this direction. Perhaps, in the future, others would not have to experience such pain. I tossed the article on my desk and closed my eyes. It was another late night with inadequate sleep and not enough time with the family. I hadn't talked with my brothers in days. It was a life out of balance.

In the midst of my folly, I reminisced about her, our times together, and a mini-event that seemed oddly related to all this . . .

After my parents' divorce, when I was eight, I remember walking with my mother and four brothers across a busy street in the Bronx. We were on our way to a counseling session at the Jewish Family Service, a social work organization dedicated to helping troubled Jewish families in the area. Our counselor was a portly, middle-aged woman, named Ms. Katzenburg.

As we crossed the street, my four brothers ran ahead, laughing, playing, making a game of beating the traffic light, poking and pushing one another, the usual antics. I ran with them, but then retreated, realizing we had left our mother. I ran back to her, held her hand, and crossed the street with her. I stayed with her the rest of the way, until we reached the familiar white brick building on Boston Road, housing the Jewish Family Service.

Ms. Katzenburg interviewed us in a room with a see-through mirror behind which sat a group of social workers and therapists who were observing us. It was quite a scene for the brothers, who thought it was slick and high-tech, something out of "Man from U.N.C.L.E.," a popular spy series on TV at the time. There was a microphone in the middle of the room, the large one-way mirror, and a gaggle of people, invisible to us, watching and listening to our every word.

In the course of the interview, my mother had brought up the incident at the busy intersection when all the boys had run ahead, leaving her. She said that I seemed to care more about her and wasn't sure how the others felt.

"Rick seems like your protector, Tilly?" Ms. Katzenburg asked.

"Yes," my mother answered.

The conversation continued and the other brothers were quick to avow their devotion to their mother, which greatly assured her, and she smiled But I didn't hear much past Ms. Katzenburg's last sentence. It was the first time I heard my relationship with my mother described in this way. From this time forward, I became my mother's protector. It was not unexpected or surprising, only the formalization of it was different, and I liked it. I didn't know how my brothers felt about it, whether they resented it or not, but they took jabs at me because of it, sneering playfully and making jokes.

But, I wore this new accolade with pride and felt suited to the role - and never relinquished it. I was permanently on hand to defend my mother's interests. If anyone ever showed disrespect to her, I confronted him. If my mother needed help around the house, I did it. If circumstances overwhelmed her, I comforted her.

I worked when I was young so I could give Mom money. I distributed ads and coupons ("circulars," we called them) for the Associated (a large supermarket nearby) on weekends and delivered groceries for tips after school. Later, I worked

in Larry's garment factory in Manhattan. It never occurred
to me **not** to give her money. Throughout the years, when I
attended college and medical school in Indiana, during my
residency in New York, my fellowship in San Francisco, and
my three years working overseas in Asia, I remained in close
contact with her – and always felt myself her protector.

With this feature of our relationship firmly established,
it was hardly ironic that Mom would come all the way to
Indiana and have her stroke. Perhaps, it was her time and
she sensed it, or perhaps it was coincidence. Either way, what
provoked guilt and anguish was that I failed to protect her.

I went to see Mom again that evening, my mind
filled with risks, tables, and algorithms for the use of
amphetamines. Yet, in her presence, it became irrelevant. Did it really matter? None of it was available for
human consumption outside of study protocols, and,
therefore, in the context of a non-teaching community
hospital, irrelevant.

"Hi, Rick." She was alert and sitting up in bed.

"Hi, Mom. Everything OK?"

The right eyebrow went up. "How's work, Rick?"
she asked.

"Fine, Mom, nothing special."

She brushed her silver hair with her right hand. She
did this all the time now. I didn't know why. I wondered if her hair bothered her for some reason, irritated her or itched or something. "No," she said when I
asked, but continued doing it anyway.

"Did anyone call you today, Mom?"

"No."

"Cliff called me," I said.

I looked over at the balloons, flowers, and get-well
cards.

"I'll bring the kids tomorrow. Maybe we'll take you
outside." My mother, a great lover of the outdoors, had
been penned in for almost two weeks. And the weather

had been perfect. It was all part of the depressing state of affairs.

In my discussions with the Rabbi, we had touched on the notion of arguing with God. The Rabbi had provided precedents: "Will you actually sweep away the just with the wicked?" Abraham asked the Lord in defending the innocent of Sodom and Gomorrah (Genesis 18:23). "Shall one man sin and You rage against the whole community?" Moses spoke in protecting the congregation of Korah (Numbers 16:22). "Why does the way of the wicked prosper?" demanded Jeremiah (Jeremiah 12:1).

Did I, too, have the right to question God? After all, tragedies of far greater magnitude occurred with unflinching regularity everyday. Misery, suffering, and death were woven into the fabric of life – and inevitable. Then there was the oddly tranquil demeanor of my mother, the victim herself – if she could maintain her composure then why not me?

"Jerry wants to call when I'm here to help you with the phone."

She nodded.

"I'll arrange the time."

"Ok."

"Rosh Hashanah is coming," I said. "We'll celebrate it here with you."

My mother looked at me as if to say, "It's alright, Rick, don't bother."

"I already spoke with the nurses," I said.

Tragedy reminded us of what was important, the shock of the event shaking us from our complacency and forcing us to examine our lives more carefully. How else might one acquire insight? Would it be wonderfully quaint to suggest that it began with speaking to God – whatever one's formulation of that elusive entity might be? Was this not the lesson behind the Biblical precedents of challenging God: to encourage us to engage Him, to confer with Him, and listen for His answer, and, hence, undertake our own inner voyage of inquiry?

I adjusted my mother's head on her pillow. "Ying will be coming."

"Don't bother Ying, she's busy," she said.

"She'll come anyway."

The tragedy of my mother's stroke was performing a kind of alchemy within me, revising me according to a different set of tables and charts. Perhaps, it was not unlike the operation it had already performed on her, instilling in her an amazing calm at the very epicenter of the turmoil. But was it driving me closer to my faith or from it?

I gazed at Mom's left hand, limp and lifeless. I caressed it and was almost surprised again to find it warm. She studied me. "It doesn't work, Rick," she said without sarcasm.

Was it a cosmic "rolling of the dice" that brought this sadness into our lives, or part of God's plan unfolding? Was it the hand of a loving God guiding us in the direction of wisdom or the natural course of a well-known disease process? Had God ceased to be a dynamic force in human history, stepping back, after the destruction of the Temple, to observe humanity work out its own salvation?

Or had God taken a different tact, withdrawing instead to the sphere of the human soul, guiding and teaching us when we chose to listen? If God no longer unleashed plagues or parted waters, did that not imply that He was also no longer responsible for the litany of tragedies that befell us? I did not want to believe that He had abandoned us.

"Any surgeries, today, Rick?" Mom asked.

"Tonsils, lumps, and bumps."

The experience of my mother's stroke had triggered many questions; it had also reawakened old memories. These rekindled a fresh awareness of the power of that most early of attachments, that of mother and child. I was flooded with images and sensations of those early years converging into a sweeping mosaic that resonated with a surprisingly joyous quality of love and dependence. I looked at those youthful memories through the prism of my middle years, which did not diminish them. I felt again as a young boy, deeply attached to his mother.

"The office OK, Rick?"

"Yeah, fine, Ma," I said.

The calm I now felt seemed the work of God. My nervous wrangling about receptors, excitatory potentiation, cerebral metabolism, and the like, receded for now. I stared across the chasm separating me from my mother and said nothing, the eloquence of silence quite satisfactory. I allowed God to continue His handiwork on her and on me, loathe at this time to argue with Him.

It was early fall in the Bronx, slightly brisk but still pleasant. It was a Saturday, and we were playing "Kick-the-Can." This was not a particularly wild street game like "Ringoleevio" or "Johnny-on-the-Pony." It was more low key with only occasional moments of high drama – mainly when the last kid holding out came bolting out of nowhere to kick the can and free his compatriots, thus launching a new cycle of running and hiding. The other element of drama was the streets themselves.

Josiah was playing with us, a black kid, the son of the new "super" (superintendent) of our building, Mr. Powell. Mr. Powell had two daughters, two other sons, and Josiah, who was about seven. He was the first black kid we had ever known. He was also the first black kid ever to come to our house. I couldn't tell if Mom liked having him in our house, but she gave him milk and cookies like my other friends. Mom thought his father was a good super, ". . . better than that lousy good for nothing we had before," she said. He wore overalls and an engineer's hat and carried a big toolbox wherever he went. He had a "southern" accent, which I had never heard before.

Cliff and I went down to his house in the basement, where supers lived, with all the boilers and heaters, to play with Josiah. It was dark and damp and the pipes ran below the ceiling, and Mr. Powell had to bend a little to keep from hitting his head. He called himself a Christian, but I never saw any pictures or crosses like the Puerto Ricans had. I guessed he was a different kind of Christian than the Puerto Ricans who were Catholics. "Thou shalt have no graven images, young man," he said when I mentioned it. He laughed in that deep, funny voice of his.

I did not remember seeing Josiah kick the can, but I knew that he did, because he was the only one left. Everyone was yelling excitedly as he ran towards the can, hoping he would "free" us so we could run and hide again. Then I heard the sound of him kicking the can, a good, strong kick, and watched the can hurtling through the air, landing on the sidewalk and rolling onto the grass. We ran, whooping like banshees, freed from our "prison" now to continue the game.

As we darted across the street, I remember seeing the diminutive Josiah running between two parked cars and hence unseen by oncoming traffic. In the periphery of my vision, I saw a blue convertible with the hood down cruising up the street and crossing the point between the two-parked cars a split second after Josiah dashed into the street. The worst part was not the sight of Josiah flying through the air and hitting the asphalt but the sound – the awful sound of bone cracking as the car struck his head. When little Josiah landed, he picked himself up, staggered to the sidewalk and fell down. He lay there, bleeding from his fractured head, dark pools forming around him.

There was panic, grown men and women screaming, grabbing their faces, pulling their hair, writhing as if in agony. "Ohmigod, Ohmigod!" one black man shouted, running up the street. *A crowd gathered, too stunned to know what to do, to pick him up, or even console him, the sight of so young a child wounded so gravely, too terrible to behold and comprehend.*

In the midst of the chaos, a dark haired woman in a white sweater appeared. I didn't recognize her at first. She was panicked like everyone else but gathered herself. She pushed through the crowd and immediately cradled Josiah in her arms, pressing his bleeding skull to her chest. She stood up and shouted commands, her voice galvanizing the throng. Someone produced a towel and wrapped it around Josiah's head. Another wiped his face and comforted him. This woman, my mother, I now realized, shouted for an ambulance, and someone yelled down from a second floor window, "We just called 'em, lady, they're on their way."

I watched my mother carry Josiah off, his ebony skin pressed against her white sweater stained with blood. She took him to his home in the basement, comforting him, talking to him, not sure if he was awake or even alive but speaking anyway, controlling the bleeding, while his father, Mr. Powell, looked on, his eyes wide with fear. Then we heard the siren. An ambulance drove up and workers took Josiah from Mom's arms.

I heard nothing about Josiah afterwards. I had no idea what became of him but ten days later, there was a knock on the door. Cliff and I ran to answer it. It was one of Josiah's older sisters – and Josiah himself. He was standing next to her, head bandaged, but smiling. They were both out of breath from having run up the stairs. The sister asked if my mother was in. When Mom came to the door, Josiah embraced her. Mr. Powell soon lumbered up the stairs with the rest of his clan.

"Thank you, Mrs. Moss, faw savin' mah boy," he said almost tearfully. Mom smiled self-consciously. Each of the other children embraced Mom and thanked her. Soon, we were playing with Josiah just like before. And Mom saved that white sweater stained with Josiah's blood.

- 26 -

He cut obliquely along the side of the neck, following the contour of the muscle, which quickly came into view. He inserted the retractor and handed it to the nurse. She grasped it and pulled, exposing the gossamer tissues, within which resided the great vessels, hidden within the downy covering. He spread and divided the feathery layers, unveiling, first, a thin walled blue structure. It was ominous in a way, the jugular vein, corpulent and throbbing, transporting gallons of blood from the brain each day, but this was not our objective. He placed a vein retractor around the pudgy thing and handed it to me. Further dissection just below it revealed something else – a whitish, pulsating, cord-like structure, lean and muscular, more foreboding than the vein, and far more significant, for this was the carotid artery, which supplied blood to the brain.

I was assisting my colleague, Don Vennekotter, a vascular surgeon. It occurred to me yesterday to speak with him – indirectly – about my mother – and make an odd request.

"You can prevent strokes?" I had asked yesterday.

"Yes, those arising from carotid artery disease."

"With surgery?"

"Yes. Carotid endarterectomy," he had answered.

"You remove the plaque from the vessel?"

"Right."

"And then they're fine?"

"Yes, usually."

"How much blockage before you recommend surgery?"

"Seventy percent."

"How do you tell?"

"Ultrasound."

"That's it?"

"Yep."

"What about medical management afterwards?" I had asked.

"Aspirin."

This was extraordinary. I had known about the benefits of aspirin as everyone did, but hearing it in the context of my mother's illness made it so much more cogent. Good ole aspirin, a fixture in everyone's medicine cabinet for generations, now no longer just drab headache medication, but one of our chief armaments against the great scourges of modern life, strokes and heart attacks. But that alone wasn't what provoked me. Rather, it was the existence of an orderly and effective sequence for preventing an insidious disease process beyond just wishful thinking or prayer.

"Patients with partial blockage of the carotid are at higher risk for having a stroke?" I had asked.

"Yes."

"How so?"

"The plaque eventually blocks the carotid or little bits may break off and enter the circulation."

"So you're preventing disability and saving lives?"

"Yes," he had answered casually.

I must have appeared astonished because he looked at me strangely. He knew of my mother's illness but was unaware of the mood swings and failures I had experienced because of it. In his world, strokes were common and treatable (or, at least, preventable). He had said so; he had informed me of the data supporting it, without hesitation. It had the full blessings of medical science and was not relegated to the domain of speculation or prayer. Here, conjecture and guesswork had no role. There were few points of uncertainty. Instead, there were precise indications and clear directives to action – surgical action. It may have applied only to the 20 percent of strokes arising from carotid artery disease, but this was still significant. Stroke, it turned out, *could* be subdued; one could anticipate it and strike preemptively. For reasons both vague and compelling, I asked if I could assist him in surgery.

By now, Don had fully exposed the carotid artery. He had carefully swept the digastric muscle and the hypoglossal nerve superiorly. He identified the vagus nerve below. The appearance of the carotid lower down in the neck was normal. As one combed upward, however, the vessel, overtaken by plaque, became increasingly misshapen and knotty, consistent with my expectations of a sinister process.

Don placed tourniquets and clamps on the vessel above and below the level of the plaque. He then cut right through the wall of the artery and into the plaque, exposing the disgusting thing for everyone to see – the accretions of fat and fibrin, the undigested stumps, the globules of grease, the gnarled, bark like irregularities where silken, glossy surfaces were the norm, the knobs of matted, craggy material that narrowed the vessel to a finite pinhole – and offended any sensibility of function and beauty. He continued filleting the vessel like a fish, exposing the inner skeleton of the plaque, thickest at the bifurcation and then tapering off modestly beyond.

"Did the patient get the heparin?" Don asked.

"Yes, Doctor," the nurse answered.

"Hand me the clamp."

With this, he began shelling out the plaque, stripping the inside of the vessel like a chestnut. Once removed, the lumen of the vessel was surprisingly smooth.

"Saline," Don requested.

I irrigated the open vessel with the solution, removing any remaining pieces of matter or debris.

"Shunt." He fit the little tube into the two ends of the divided artery, released clamps, and, amazingly, restored circulation to the brain.

"Patch."

The nurse handed him a slender Dacron ribbon, which he trimmed and inserted into the defect.

"Six-0 Prolene."

He began meticulously suturing it, tiny stitches methodically placed, carefully approximating the synthetic strip to the vessel wall and increasing its diameter, a marriage of the artificial and the natural. "It's treated with protein so it doesn't leak," he mentioned to me by way of instruction.

It fascinated me, both philosophically and technically. The territory was quite familiar to me, having visited it hundreds of times, but for different reasons – generally the removal of tumors. In my world, the carotid was sacred, never to be transgressed, always minded with the utmost respect. But here was a *deliberate* assault on it, splicing and shelling it, and, as if to add further insult, repairing it with a synthetic ribbon, an embarrassment to so regal a structure, yet vital and life sustaining.

With the final stitches joining patch and artery, he removed the shunt and released the clamps. It leaked like a sieve. "Gelfoam and thrombin," Don requested. He placed this over the artery and applied pressure to control the bleeding. "Give the Protamine." (This to reverse the anticoagulant effects of the heparin given previously.) The leaking around the patch gradually slowed, the hybrid, reconstituted vessel intact and patent – and free flowing – providing oxygen rich blood to the brain.

"Let's close," Don said.

I understood the sources of my eccentric joy. It was ever so redemptive (and preemptive). Stroke was not invincible. The medical sciences could triumph after all. It was a pleasure to see the directness of the repair. No annoying discussions or research protocols, no amphetamines, TPA, or bat saliva. Here, there was straightforward diagnosis and intervention with good outcomes. Here there was restitution and repair, and a solid upward trajectory.

I quietly paid homage to this elegant procedure, the carotid endarterectomy, and the skill of my colleague, who, perhaps, unknowingly, had done *me* a great service, as well as his patient. It was to this resurgence that I clung, looking for signs of hope. That my mother's illness had profoundly affected me was obvious; that someone else's restoration could relieve me was unexpected. Don was placing the final stitches.

"Thank you, Don," I told him with surprising urgency and enthusiasm.

The most important room in our crowded little apartment in the Bronx was the bathroom. This single indispensable sanctuary in the house made life possible, and we regarded it with proper reverence. There were six of us and so the presence of a single such chamber presented formidable obstacles, most notably in the morning. It began at 7 a.m. when Mom awakened us. We could hear her in the kitchen, opening the refrigerator and pouring the orange juice. We could hear her jiggling the bottle of vitamins and laying each one down on the washing machine. Then, she walked down the long hallway leading to the two bedrooms where we slept.

"Rise and shine," she said pleasantly. She walked into the bedroom and laid the glasses of orange juice on the dresser

along with the vitamins. "Time to get up," she said, and by now, we were beginning to stir. We put the little yellow pills in our mouths and drank the juice. Then came the scramble for the bathroom.

Because Larry was oldest, he went first. The bathroom door closed, the little hook latched, and the rest of us stood in line, impatiently waiting to urinate. Often, there were clashes over who went next. There was much dancing and squirming, not to mention gnashing of teeth. My mother came up with a solution.

Coke bottles were returnable, worth two cents a bottle. We saved the empties, six in a carton, and piled them next to the refrigerator. Once a week, we placed some fifty bottles into the shopping cart and returned them to the store for a buck. With the big line up at the bathroom each morning, my mother began handing out Coke bottles. We never realized how hot urine was until we watched the bottles steam up after we peed in them. We held them up and made faces on them with our fingers through the steam. Most of us were fine with one bottle, except for Jack who needed two. He filled up the first bottle, the warm yellow liquid stopping just short of overflowing and then switching quickly to the second, all of which he did with great deft.

When we each had our chance to enter the bathroom, we dumped the contents of the bottles into the toilet and rinsed them to be returned, of course. This little system devised by my mother served the family well for years. It would, no doubt, have broken down completely had we had sisters.

So, each morning after Larry locked the bathroom door, the rest of us lined up doing our jigs, while Mom rushed to the kitchen and grabbed empty Coke bottles. We didn't mind waiting to brush our teeth. But we were happy to have the empty bottles when we had to take a leak.

- 27-

I visited my mother that evening. I felt as if I had not seen her in a while, which was foolish since I had been there last night. But such were the peculiarities of perception, distorted as they were by the vagaries of my obsessions and conceits. Life visited far greater calamities upon humanity than this, yet it still consumed me. The taking of a loved one in so ruthless a manner, the flippancy and impertinence of disease – barging in on an otherwise satisfactory existence.

Life did that though. It acted independently of our interests, as if to remind us of its destructive talents. That it was September, a splendid month, did not matter. That the High Holy days were approaching was immaterial. That this was my mother was irrelevant. It was the contempt for human affairs, however trivial they may be, that provoked me. But who better, after all, than a physician, to understand the fickle nature of life given the continuous stream of disasters that passed through his office every day?

Such considerations did not seem to consume my mother's energies. She looked up, obviously fatigued, but managed a smile. It had been more than two weeks since the stroke.

"Hi Rick," she said with slurred speech. She appeared no different and maintained the same calm demeanor. She was lying on her back, the head of bed elevated, bedrails up, NG tube in place, and the creamy white liquid streaming in through her nose. She was on a soft diet, but eating very little. A Foley catheter was present, the tubing and bag off to the side. The TV was silent. A nurse had arranged the flowers, cards, and balloons carefully on the shelf. Nothing had changed. Her left side still cleaved to the right, a useless appendage limply hanging on. It was still "living" in a sense, sustained by circulation – but numb and paralyzed.

Only the right half still lived in the true sense of the word. Could the left side encroach upon it, I wondered, more than by the mere additional burden it represented, its weight and lack of function, but, rather, by evil intent, sinister purpose, or direct aggression somehow? Was it not a fundamental tenet that life did not thrive in the presence of death, that death inevitably encroached and consumed it?

"You look good Rick," Mom said, again smiling. She was tired, bedridden and incapacitated, but she showed no remorse. Rather, it appeared she had used her stroke as a fulcrum with which to jerk herself into higher orbits. It was almost a parody to hear her compliment me or to inquire how I was, so unlikely under the circumstances. Yet, perhaps, this was only my petty understanding of it. She had shown herself very resourceful in the past, and perhaps this was merely the latest such example. What was unusual and completely unprecedented was her tranquility. This launched me into ever expanding spheres of metaphysical contemplation.

"You look good, too," I answered.

She looked at me, raising her eyebrow, suggesting she did not need to hear such rubbish. Actually, she did look good. Her face was smooth, her cheeks pink, and her eyes clear. Her silver hair was combed back. She wore no make up. The stroke had impounded her flesh but not her soul. She was much too calm to say that and did not seem a prisoner.

I told her of yesterday's adventure in the operating room with Dr. Vennekotter. She seemed intrigued. This, too, was uncharacteristic. Generally, she was proud of the accomplishments of her sons but did not revel in the details. Success for her boys was adequate for her. Yet here she was inquiring into points of academic interest, the appearance of the plaque, how readily it shelled out, even the chemical composition of the offensive material, and whether diet could alter it. She asked about the likelihood of success and how quickly such patients were discharged.

In the discussion, I sensed no envy or resentment, no self-pity for the failure to prevent her calamity, only an unlikely curiosity that demonstrated itself despite the physical constraints of her condition. Her speech remained slurred, but if she took her time, it was comprehensible. She fatigued easily but maintained her interest.

I did most of the talking, which was nothing new. In fact, I had always enjoyed regaling my mother with my feats: whom I had bested in debate, what outlandish project I had completed, or which obscure locale I had operated in during my travels. Whatever subject I was expounding, she seemed prepared to listen. For me, the joy of my mother had always been this: her willingness to indulge me interminably.

Most of the time though she only listened, an occasional nod to indicate her understanding and endorsement. During such discourses, I could better clarify my thoughts. I could not recall her cutting me off prematurely. Her ready ear was something I expected and appreciated. What enhanced my appreciation was the sense that she enjoyed listening. Yet it was rare for her to query me. But here, sickly, her powers severely diminished, she displayed a quixotic inquisitiveness. I enjoyed this new aspect of her personality.

"How is Ying?" she asked. This question startled me, given the frostiness of their relationship. She generally asked me about the kids but not Ying. But here she specifically asked about her.

"She's fine," I answered.

"I'd like to see her." Again, I wondered at the bizarre alchemy at work within her.

"OK," I answered curiously.

I glanced at the Jewish star hanging from her necklace and the jade pendant Ying had given her behind it. She noticed but said nothing.

"Jerry wants me to call when I'm here to help with the phone."

She nodded.

"I'll bring the kids over."

She nodded again.

"How's your swallowing?"

The nurse's notes were not encouraging: 150 cc intake by mouth over the last 24 hours. The heretofore-straightforward manipulation of a bolus of food from the oral cavity to the back of the throat and the subsequent swallow was altogether too difficult for her now. She had spent time in the chair. She needed three nurses to move her – with the Hoyer lift. They turned her twice. They had bathed and given her mouth care.

"Did physical therapy come by?" I asked.

She nodded. Here she began to fade – as if any allusion to her body depressed her. She looked tired, her eyes drifting.

The nurse's aide had changed her linens. Perianal and catheter care given. The speech therapist had been in to see her. She had tried pureed food with thick liquids but minimal intake.

"What happened to the NG tube?" I asked in reference to a note indicating that a nurse had reinserted it. No answer. I hoped she had not pulled it. They called Dr. Regan and he ordered a new one and an X-ray to check placement. I glanced at her again. The NG tube was taped in and functioning, a new one apparently placed. She was OK. I saw also that she was almost asleep. This remained the dominant reality.

The brief interludes of attentiveness and conversation were like ephemeral bubbles that burst quickly. She had stamina for perhaps 15 minutes. Beyond that, the familiar pattern followed: nods of the head, glazed eyes, disinterest, and sleep. Timing was essential. In the morning, even this measly scrap was impossible. I felt the gathering winds and the bad omens. I could not escape my premonitions, her transient moments of lucency notwithstanding.

I found myself praying to God and simultaneously speculating on His presence. I did not expect or even contemplate asking for physical cure, only something to weaken the curtain enfolding *me*. I felt the deepening wound revealing itself, the inability to hear myself.

I called upon Him, now, as I had called upon the mother who slept. Prayer poured out spontaneously. Would The Name, *HaShem,* hear me? Would the *Ruach Hakodesh,* the Holy Presence, heed me? I sought Him as an *immanent* presence, not the transcendent God of history. Was that too much? I had become dutiful in my prayer obligations, submitting to the obligatory quotient of worship. I reasoned that I was at liberty to seek his aid. I did not feel awkward in doing so.

My mother had worked herself into a deep sleep. The conversation thusly ended, I sat with her silently. I prayed for her healing – and mine.

> Save us, divine Ruler, when we call;
> Make me to know the path of life,
> the fullness of joy in thy presence,
> at Thy right hand eternal bliss.

Rosh Hashanah was a legal holiday in New York because there were so many Jews in the city. All the other major Jewish holidays were legal holidays, too, including Yom Kippur, Sukkoth, and Passover. Despite the sizeable Jewish presence in New York, the holidays and other Jewish events that took place there, I recognized we still lived in a Christian world. The signs and symbols of that larger world were unavoidable.

In school, we heard about Christian holidays, and most kids in school were Christian. There were many churches in the neighborhood, far more than synagogues. When walking with Christian friends, I noticed some of them crossing themselves or kneeling when passing a church, which was often. Many homes I visited had crucifixes.

As a child, I was at turns resentful of the dominant Christian culture, feeling it as something foreign and overwhelming, even, perhaps, hostile. At the time, I had no idea how tiny and vulnerable the Jewish people were in the world, as the Jewish population in New York, although a minority was still formidable. Nor did I as yet know of the long chronicle of Christian antipathy and persecution against the Jews. Rather, it was more a visceral reaction to something unfamiliar to me. It was during Rosh Hashanah, however, years ago when an event occurred that transformed that early suspicion of Christianity into something more florid and substantial.

It was mid-September on the first day of Rosh Hashanah, a flawless day, and I was walking home from the synagogue with my mother and Cliff. Jerry was ahead of us with a friend. We wore our finest clothes and our yarmulkes, and Mom was holding our hands.

I saw some kids from another neighborhood riding bikes. They were tough looking kids and rowdy. They were cutting in and out of traffic, riding between parked cars, jumping curves, shouting brazenly, as if to spite the sanctity of our holiday. I felt my mother's grip tighten. There were four kids, teenagers, perhaps, and they charged past us on their bikes toward Jerry. I wanted to run ahead, but my mother restrained me as she quickened her gait. *The four kids rode up the street to the corner opposite Jerry. They continued yelling and carrying on, tossing out an occasional obscenity, as if to mock us. There was a garbage can nearby, which they rummaged through, to find some bottles. They played with them, laughing, teasing, and gesturing with them in threatening ways. I let go of Mom's hand and hastened towards Jerry.*

"Ricky," Mom called, again trying to restrain me, but I ignored her this time. Jerry was still talking with a friend, unaware of the presence of the four young hooligans gathered across the street. I saw their angry faces; then I heard those fateful words. "Christ killers!" they shouted shockingly. Whom were they addressing? I was confused. The answer was forthcoming. "Hey, you damn Christ killers," they screamed, looking at Jerry and his friend. Jerry, a Christ killer? Jerry lifted his head towards the kids, hearing them at last.

"Jerry," I yelled, running towards him. I heard Mom scream Jerry's name, too, as she ran with Ronnie in tow. Then I heard a crash, as a bottle shattered at Jerry's feet, and then another crash. Jerry started running when a bottle caught him in the mouth. More bottles flew and crashed around us. I saw Jerry's bloody face, the shattered glass on the sidewalk, and picked the biggest shard and hurled it back

My mother grabbed me, saying, "Stop it, Ricky, they're too big!" I screamed, "No, I hate them, I'll get them." I broke free long enough to see them jumping on their bikes and racing off, scornful and laughing, repeating again the epithet that I despised and did not understand: "Christ killers!" they shouted. I yelled back, "I never killed Christ, I never met Christ! I don't know who he is!" They disappeared in the maze of streets, and I never saw them again.

A crowd gathered around us, helping my mother who was holding a handkerchief to Jerry's bleeding mouth. She comforted him as she cursed under her breath. "Damn bastards," she said. When she lifted the stained handkerchief from his face, she looked and gasped.

"Oh God in heaven," she shouted, "his teeth!" She began weeping, "Look what they did to his teeth!" She held Jerry's face to her chest. I saw a front upper tooth cracked obliquely, a jagged, bloody stump. "Find the piece," she screamed.

We mindlessly obeyed, as if it would matter, scouring the sidewalk, brushing the glass with our hands, looking vainly for tiny fragments of tooth enamel amidst the broken glass. Mom cried and cursed again. The incident was much worse now because of this, because she had no money to repair it, and because it would be a daily reminder of the event. "He had such beautiful teeth," Mom cried aloud, holding Jerry close to her, who wept but seemed comforted by her. She held the stained handkerchief over his mouth, cursing as we trudged home.

- 28 -

I was sitting in my living room thinking about forgiveness and how one received it. I had felt contemptible all day. I made it through the workday, the weight of my ill humor upon me. I did not know how to escape. How long would I be able to put up the charade and disguise myself as a physician, husband, and father? The illness was odious and unassailable, like an unclean presence. In my life as bourgeois man, I could scarcely endure these forays into meaningless introspection. The stroke of my mother was afflicting me again, an open wound that would not heal. Yet, were my efforts all in vain? Had I not taken measures to purge myself?

My brother Jerry had called earlier. He wanted to know how Mom was doing, and then turned aggressive.

"Why isn't she progressing?" he asked, as if stroke were the same as a sprained ankle. I took offense, as if he were blaming me. But he was right. I had already resigned myself to her condition. My excursions into the world of stroke literature seemed more to conceal my hopelessness than anything. Therapy was the answer, not experimental medicines. Yet I defended myself to him.

"Not everything has a happy ending," I said. He brushed aside my pathetic rebuttal.

"But what are you doing to improve her condition?" he pressed with callous disregard for my feebleness.

"Everything I can."

"It's not enough."

"How about kissing my butt," I said stupidly.

But on further reflection, he was right.

I called Regan, still ringing from my brother's criticisms, and asked how she was doing. "Real slow, Rick, she's not moving at all."

"What can we do?" I asked.

"Well, I don't know. I think she's doing about as well as she can." He paused and then suggested I contact TriStateRehab out of Evansville. "They're doing innovative things; even some work with robots."

This excited me. I made an appointment. They would evaluate her next week. I felt relieved with this, enjoying some sense of achievement. This dissipated quickly though when I realized that nothing would come of it. I had become dense like my brother, thinking I could make a difference.

But couldn't I? The conflict of motives quickly mutated into a sense of futility. I despised my incompetence. I could barely move or take a step. I had merely transformed into an effective actor, maintaining a facade I could no longer bear. I was still at war with myself, but I was also growing weary of the endless self-recrimination and ineffectiveness.

My wife had come in before, as had my children, and again the charade continued. I had dispatched them as politely as I could. I had eaten dinner, even taken a walk with my children. Now alone, I stared at the four walls and painted ceiling of my kitchen, a sky blue with puffy tufts of white clouds, almost transporting. I got lost in these apparitions, the ghosts of my thoughts bellowing, the absurd expressions of clouds whirling about meaninglessly, happy to be alone.

I then acted out of desperation. I took out my yarmulke, a beautiful Sephardic style headpiece, green and red, with golden decorative embroidery around it in soothing shapes and patterns, and small luminous buttons sewn in that made it almost glitter. I put it on. I delighted in the sensation, its weight and presence upon my head, feeling somehow affected by it, a slight dusting of sanctity that soothed me. Then I wondered about the nature of forgiveness.

That I needed absolution was apparent. I required it in order to breathe. I could not, however, burden my mother with this. For now, I would have to seek it from the Holy One, blessed be He. Such an enterprise implied belief in a God who cared enough to listen; a God that could decipher me from the multitude of others seeking him out; a God who could interpret my pleas, winnow mine from the countless others, decipher the legitimate from the profane, and then decide to intercede.

How all this transpired I could only guess. What organs of sense, cognition, and function enabled God to hear, construe, and act was beyond knowing. What the logistics of such interaction, not to mention the handling of the millions upon millions of other similar desperate appeals occurring each moment, was unfathomable.

I simply followed the traditions, which were as accessible to me as they were to anyone willing to suspend judgment. I was quite secure in my belief in the mastery of science, quite comfortable within the stale doctrines of logic and analysis. Yet there had always been that thread planted in me years ago by none other than my mother, that slender filament she had drawn that wound me to a field beyond reason, a domain beyond dissection, and into the realm of faith. I was seeking forgiveness, wounded by my failures, and the unhappy lot of my mother.

I visited Mom in the morning, tempting fate, because I knew that was not her good time. The therapists, however, came in the morning, and I wanted to watch them, remembering my conversation with Jerry. Were they doing all they could? How was she progressing? Was I doing enough? She was already up in the chair when I walked in; the Hoyer lift that had moved her was sitting just outside the room. She looked better sitting up, her eyes more clear and alert. She acknowledged me with a raised eyebrow. The same two therapists were working on her left hand: Sara, the sergeant physical therapist, who never smiled, and Roberta, the matronly and much friendlier occupational therapist. The two still found it necessary to pool their efforts in a single session.

The therapists acknowledged me. They were doing more occupational therapy, which meant upper extremity, to encourage Mom to move her fingers, hands, and arms to perform specific tasks like lifting a cup, writing a letter, or feeding herself. Her right hand, of course, presented no problem. For the left, it was futile. There was no movement. I consoled myself with the knowledge that perhaps such activity served to rekindle the ancient memories of movement, as the therapists had explained before.

I tried to smile at the dismal performance, maintaining the facade for my mother's sake. She appeared listless.

"Come on, Matilda," Roberta said, trying to salvage something. They were bending the wrist forward and backward, all movements fully passive, Mom unable to contribute a smidgen. They asked her to make a fist and spread her fingers. Nothing. Perhaps, if Jerry saw this, he would be less ambitious. They turned to the leg and foot, with similarly disappointing results. They plied their craft diligently working as little drones, unsmiling and methodical. Roberta occasionally brightened up the atmosphere with a comment or chuckle.

When they finished, I inquired privately with the therapists how long Mom would be eligible for Skilled Care. We were nearly three weeks past the stroke and I knew time was running out. Regan had informed me that Medicare would stop covering Skilled Care unless the therapists demonstrated some progress. I wanted to know their impressions.

"She's not doing much," Roberta said sadly.

I nodded at the obvious.

"We can keep her around a while longer. Maybe she'll improve."

This I felt to be unrealistic but gratefully accepted this tiny morsel of hope.

"Is that indicated in your notes?"

"Yes," said Roberta, "but there are limits to what we can say to justify her staying."

Her tone sparked the broker in me. "So how long are we talking about?"

"Seven days. Ten at best," she said.

It was actually more than I expected. A grim thought resurfaced; if she did not improve, I would soon have to contemplate a nursing home.

I sat down next to my mother who was still awake. She did not seem perturbed.

"How do you feel?"

She shrugged, raised her right eyebrow, and said, "I'm OK, Rick. How are you?"

The question seemed comical, but I was growing used to it. "Fine, Ma."

"How'd that patient do?" Mom asked.

"Which one?"

"The carotid patient."

This, also, remained odd to me, her uncanny curiosity about that case. "Dr. Vennekotter told me he was going home today," I answered.

She smiled. "Good."

"I want to speak with Larry," she said, completely changing the topic. I nodded.

"I'll arrange it."

She smiled, but I could see she was drifting. I let it go. Morning time was sleep time for her now, she who had always been so active in the mornings. I wanted to tell her about Rosh Hashanah but decided against it. It interested me that she wanted to speak with Larry.

I watched her eyes close. I glanced at the oblique scar on her forehead. The room was quiet, the curtain drawn between her and her roommate who was also sleeping. Slumber had overtaken the room. I merged with it, allowing my thoughts to wander.

I worried about her but less so in her presence. The fog of gloom evaporated when I was with her. I agonized over the uncertain realities awaiting us, particularly if she failed to improve. Yet, sitting here with her, the edges of my anxiety softened. Her serenity, I realized, was a balm for me, a blessing. Perhaps, it was intentional.

She fell ill here, appeared destined to stay here, showed no signs of meaningful recovery, yet was an oasis of calm, as if she knew where she was going. She also seemed to be making overtures. She wanted to talk with Ying and now with Larry. I was unready for the logical conclusions, still hoping to bring her home, away from shadows and phantoms, and from my dark imaginings.

I watched her, observing the light movement of her chest, the warm air entering and exiting her lungs, sustaining her as she slept, she adrift in an obscure enclosure, communing with her dreams, understanding better than I what awaited her. I wondered foolishly if she knew all this, if she could see the future. Had she even chosen the setting of her ordeal, perhaps of her end? And this thought worried me greatly.

*"In the seventh month, on the first day of the month, you
shall observe a holy day;
a memorial proclaimed with the blast of the horn, a holy
convocation.
You shall do no servile work."*

Leviticus 23:24-25

This day became known as Rosh Hashanah, the
Jewish New Year. It began the *Yamin Noraim,* the Days
of Awe, the high holy days, the ten days of repentance.
Two traditional beliefs were associated with Rosh Hashanah that endowed it with particular religious power: that it was the anniversary of the Creation of the
world (*Yom Harat Olam*), and a Day of Judgment (*Yom
Hadin*). It marked the beginning of the ten-day period
of spiritual introspection and repentance that culminated with *Yom Kippur,* the Day of Atonement.

Intensive prayer and meditation marked the tone
of Rosh Hashanah. Acceptance of God's dominion over
the world was the prevailing theme. Then there was
the blowing of the shofar, the ram's horn. When the
shofar was sounded, one concentrated on its meaning
and gave heed to its call to repent. It hearkened back to
Sinai, when thunder engulfed the majestic mountain,
as God delivered His revelation to Moses, the time
when the Jewish people were closest to God. According to tradition, God sat in judgment of humanity on
Rosh Hashanah. Through repentance and prayer, one
moved toward reconciliation. Observant Jews recited
the penitential prayers, the *Selichot.*

Merciful God, open the heavens to prayer,
for Thine infinite mercy.
Merciful God, receive our prayers with favor,
for Thine infinite mercy.
Merciful God, bring upon us a good year,
for Thine infinite mercy.

Merciful God, turn Thine indignation from us,
for Thine infinite mercy.
Merciful God, let us not go empty from Thy presence,
for Thine infinite mercy.

". . . the tenth day of this seventh month is the
Day of Atonement.
It shall be a holy convocation to you,
and you shall afflict your souls.
You shall do no work throughout that day,
for it is a day of atonement;
it is a law for all time. . . ."

Leviticus 16:30-31

The Day of Atonement, Yom Kippur, was the last chance before the gates were closed, and God completed His judgment. It was observed with a complete fast (". . . you shall afflict your souls . . ."), prayer, and reflection. Yom Kippur was the culmination of the penitential efforts of the High Holy Days.

Our Father and King, we have sinned before Thee.
Our Father and King, bring us back through perfect
repentance.
Our Father and King, grant our prayer, if not for our
own merit, then for Thine own sake.
Our Father and King, accept our prayer with favor
and mercy.
Our Father and King, turn us not away empty from
Thy presence.

At the end of Yom Kippur, the final blast of the shofar was sounded. We have returned in repentance to a moral and decent life. With God's blessing, we are cleansed and reconciled before Him.

I took the kids to visit Nona. It was Saturday, just two days before Rosh Hashanah. It was another impeccable day, the sky cloudless and brilliant. I wanted to take my mother out to enjoy the day as she always had. But her condition had fixed her within the four walls of her hospital room, not once going out since the dreaded event. She had always been passionate about the world of nature, of communing with the elements, she who had sought to paint the sky.

She did not greet my wishes with enthusiasm. It was the morning, yes, not her best time.

She looked at me with apathy. I hid my disappointment and prevailed upon her. The kids assisted. They said, "C'mon, Nona." She smiled at them, their clean, fresh faces, fragrant and appealing, their infectious sweetness lifting her.

The nurses began the process. There were three of them. They shifted her to her left and slipped the canvas belt beneath her. They pressed a button on the panel of the Hoyer lift and the mechanism engaged, lifting her up toward the reclining wheel chair. Another button and the apparatus lowered her into it. The nurses performed flawlessly, a familiar routine.

My mother, too, seemed inured to it, indifferent and only slightly disgusted. I realized what a terrible burden this was, and my insistence that she join us seemed selfish. Was it better to let her lay? She had already accepted her fate. Was I now forcing her to do things she no longer cared about, whatever her prior passions may have been, to soothe myself?

I realized I could not begin to fathom her thoughts and wishes. She had shifted into other realms. She would never tell what she knew or how she felt. She would not impose it upon us. She must have labored against the grim recognition of the realities of her condition, of her destiny, and the daily humiliations. Perhaps, she wondered why I did not see what she saw; so I would not burden her, and she would not have to tell me. She would not have to give shape and substance to the pernicious thoughts by forming them into utterances. And why should I augment the misery by imposing this arduous charade of normalcy upon her?

The nurses moved her into the hallway and I took over the helm of the wheelchair. I moved her down the corridor to the elevator, pressed the button, and waited. The children stood on either side of her, grasping her hand.

"It's beautiful, Ma. I thought you'd like to go out," I said.

She made no real gesture but seemed to acquiesce. The kids looked at her and she smiled valiantly at them. With her right hand, she caressed Arielle's face. The elevator door opened and we descended. I pushed her down the long hall toward the exit. Hospital workers greeted us. We turned right at the corner and exited the sliding doors and then outside. I positioned her by a bench in the shade and we sat down.

The day was exquisite – a jewel of a day and yet my mother did not seem impressed. Rather, she was indifferent. I asked the kids to tell her what they did this week. This seemed to animate her. After a time, the kids grew impatient. I was yearning only for the most pedestrian of things, to go for a walk and enjoy the day, but that was all distant now, like relics from another age.

"Isn't it beautiful, Ma?" I said.

She nodded with little conviction.

"I wish we could go somewhere," I said. She stared at me as if I were dim. Then she said something unexpected.

"Rick, you're gonna have to get used to this."

I looked at her. She seemed to be chiding me. I assumed, of course, she was referring to her condition. Undaunted, I stupidly continued. "Do you like being outside?" I asked.

"It is beautiful," she offered half-heartedly, more to pacify me.

"Rosh Hashanah is coming," I announced.

I was happy beyond measure for the little smile this seemed to elicit. I realized I did not want to let her go. I wanted to engage her in the rituals and rhythms of life as we had always known them, and would go as far as she would allow me.

"How is the practice, Rick?" she asked.

"Good."

"Busy?"

"Uh huh."

My mother carried on as if nothing was wrong.

"Cliff's coming out next week."

She smiled at this. That her kids still loved her enough to visit was satisfaction for her.

"It's odd that all this happened out here, huh, Ma?"

To this, my mother said nothing.

"I'm arranging for you to see TriStateRehab. They're good."

She nodded.

My mother had disappointed me in the years after our childhood. She had remained set in her role as mother even after we were out of the house. I encouraged her to develop older vintage talents, such as painting, or to pursue areas of interest that I knew she had, but she refused. I suggested Biblical or Judaic Studies or a foreign language or perhaps an instrument. I reviewed course materials and catalogues with her. She did nothing. She was stuck in one mode and refused to listen.

Her divorce with Dad, I realized, had trapped her, even decades after the event. I criticized her for it, but to no avail. I wanted to engage her about Dad and the experience of that period, discussing years later a painful phase in our shared lives, yet she could not or would not. She grew silent, put on an enigmatic Mona Lisa smile, and looked away. She remained in many ways a child, trapped by a bitter chapter from her past.

Yet, now, I sensed she had moved past that, past many things. If anything, I was the one fixed and sealed in a box.

I glanced at my mother and suddenly realized that she was unwell. She was sweating profusely and breathing hard. Yet she said nothing. I stood up. She said in a slurred voice, "It's not your fault, Rick."

This comment shocked me. I felt some sudden sense of reprieve but then returned quickly to the trouble at hand.

"Are you OK, Mom?"

I called the kids over. "Let's get Nona inside. She's too hot."

I turned the chair and hurriedly pushed her through the sliding doors and into the hospital. The immediate gust of cool air felt good. I removed the blanket covering her and wiped the sweat from her brow. She seemed to feel better. "Are you OK, Ma?" I asked again.

She nodded.

"Let's go back up."

I wheeled her to the elevator and up to her room. The nurses took over, brought cool rags, and comforted her. She was very tired. I asked one of the nurses to check her blood pressure. It was normal. I felt relieved. She was so fragile now. She could tolerate so little.

I thought about my mother's words.

She had forgiven me, it seemed, although I had not asked for it. I thanked her silently even as I wondered what exactly she had intended.

The next day, I saw a patient of mine, someone I had known for years. She was an elderly woman with lymphoma, first discovered in the neck (by me, years before) and now in remission. She came in periodically to have me check her. She was a pleasant woman, with much good cheer. She had an attractive, elderly face, thin, and elegant, and neatly styled white hair. She was well spoken and an avid reader. We had always enjoyed discussions on a range of topics when she visited unrelated to her illness.

I examined her neck, the smooth contours interrupted only by an oblique linear scar on the left side. It was a testimonial to my brief surgical foray there while sampling an enlarged node, subsequently found to be malignant. The tumor, although advanced (stage III, the oncologist determined), was amenable to treatment. She had remained disease free, her neck still supple with no offending lumps to suggest a return of the malignancy.

I told her as before that everything looked fine. She nodded appreciatively and then – quite coincidentally (I had said nothing of my mother) – informed me with an emotional, quivering voice that her husband of more than forty years had had a stroke. She spoke in the manner of a tempest, a sudden and near violent release of painful thoughts and feelings requiring expression.

It was a devastating stroke, she said, involving the left side of the brain. It occurred a few months before. His status was that of invalid, his right side paralyzed; he was bedridden, dependent on nurses and aides for all mundane tasks and personal hygiene. I had met her husband at the time of her surgery, a handsome, vigorous man, successful in business, outgoing and athletic. He was elderly, like his wife, but the curling thick white locks, the only slightly wrinkled facial skin and energetic manner, belied his age. The two of them shared many interests, doted on their children and grandchildren, and in so many ways led a deeply satisfying life together.

"He was on Coumadin," she said. "He had atrial fibrillation, but they corrected it, and so the doctor reduced his dosage. I asked him whether we should continue the same dosage, but he said the reduced dose was OK. A few days later, he had the stroke. I was so angry," she said and began to cry.

"It affected his right side, his good side. He cannot walk or write. It damaged his cognitive function. When he reads I have to tell him to go to the next line. He doesn't understand the words. His speech is affected. He cries all the time, sudden uncontrollable outbursts, which is so unlike him. We had such wonderful times together. It is such a loss, such a terrible loss," she said.

She mentioned that the neurologist diagnosed him with *Broca's aphasia,* which affected speech centers in the dominant lobe and even though the structures of articulation (tongue, lips, larynx . . .) were intact, the patient was unable to express or interpret words. This, fortunately, my mother had been spared, her thought processes left intact.

"A month later, he had a second stroke, which weakened him further. He lost strength, couldn't stand, and became completely bedridden. He was on the full dose of Coumadin and still had the stroke," she said.

"He gets so angry, curses a lot, which is so out of character for him. He doesn't understand why he can't get better. He has even talked about committing suicide." She became very distraught. I tried to calm her. "Then he says, 'I can't do that because then I may not see you in heaven.' Then he tells me, 'I do know I love you,' and he thanks me for taking care of him."

It was amazing how riveted I was by her story, how attuned to the calamity, so obviously relevant to my own narrative. The power of her emotions, the depth of the misfortune, and the abruptness of the dislocation were all familiar themes. This, I well knew, was the harvest of stroke.

"Where is he going for rehab?" I asked.

Her answer was significant to me. "TriStateRehab. They're excellent."

"Where's he living now?"

"In Brookside."

"He can't live at home?"

"No. I tried everything, remodeled the house to accommodate him, nursing aides, family, but it was too much. He's only five minutes from home. I visit twice a day. Sometimes he tells me to go, that I need a break. He chases me away." She laughed and smiled as she thought of him. "He was always so caring."

"How does he look?"

"Like himself, still handsome. If he doesn't speak or try to do anything, you'd never know anything was wrong with him. That's what's so strange about it."

Many times since my mother's stroke, I had thought this very same thing: about the insidious nature of this disease, its clandestine but pitiless aspect.

"How are you doing?" I asked.

"Not well. I had such high hopes, so many plans for us, to travel and visit grandkids. We did so many things together. I still can't sleep, even with sleeping pills. Frankly, it's destroying me." She stood up, more to regain some measure of self-control. I handed her a tissue. "I don't know when I'll get over this, when I'll feel like myself again. I'm on tranquilizers. I just can't stand it."

She turned away from me, as if embarrassed by her emotions, she who had always been so composed. She was in the midst of her torment, roiled and beset by violent passions that she seemed unable to manage. I observed her, engaged yet analytic, empathetic but detached, the comparisons inevitable, the similarities compelling. I watched her as if watching myself, seeing my own agony replayed in altered form, all the more poignant when seeing the cruel efficiency of the disease at work in someone else. "But I have to move past this," she said. "I have to present myself better to him. It won't do for me to be a wreck when he is like this."

With this final thought, she seemed to pull herself together. She adjusted herself and smiled. I walked her out, moved by her grief, she another casualty of the great demiurge, stroke.

After the divorce, Dad remarried. But Dad still wanted to see his kids. Mom wouldn't let him. She was full of anger and rage and struck back at him with her greatest weapon – her children, whom she kept from him. The older ones, however, could travel. When she found out one day that Jack and Larry took the subway down to see him at his furniture store in Harlem, on 125th street, she went nuts. She berated them as if they had betrayed her. The two boys stared at the ground, faces buried in shame. They continued visiting him regularly though, only surreptitiously, like adulterers sneaking around. But the three youngest never saw him.

When Larry was 21, he announced that he was marrying his high school sweetheart, Helen Becker, 18, daughter of Holocaust survivors, someone more like a sister to us, whom everyone loved. This was no surprise. What was a surprise was what came next.

"I want Dad to come," Larry said.

*Mom stared at him, her face suddenly knotted up into a tight ball. "How **dare** you."*

"He's my father, and I want him to come," he repeated.

"No way he will," she said.

"It's my wedding," he said.

Mom continued gaping at him, galled by the effrontery but also incredulous that he would be foolish enough to continue down this path: "Are you a moron?" she asked.

"I want my father to come to my wedding," he responded, a slight edge in his voice.

"Over my dead body!"

"Mom, be reasonable."

"I'll give you reasonable," she said, making a fist and holding it right up to his face.

"It's **my** wedding, and he's **my** father."

"I don't care!"

"I know how you feel."

"Don't give me that bull!" she raged.

"I want him there."

"You little fool."

"Don't talk this way."

"He destroys our marriage, wrecks our family, and you want him at your wedding?" She laughed with scorn.

"Yes, **my** wedding!"

"You ingrate!"

"And Helen wants him to come." A miscalculation.

"Helen wants him to come," she said in a mocking, sneering voice. "I don't care what Helen wants!" she spat. "Or her mother. Or anyone. Do you hear me?"

"Stop it."

"You stop it, do you hear me – and you decide! Because if he comes, then I don't!" She glared at her oldest son, a surprising smile almost forming upon her lips.

Larry closed his eyes and took a breath. He relented. "Alright," he said, surrendering. He would not invite his father after all. He would not risk inviting misery into his new life for the presence of his father, the outcast. He walked away and nothing more was said.

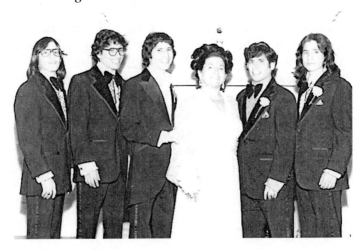

- 29 -

It was sunny and warm. I was sitting on my patio eating breakfast. The kids were playing in the woods next to my house. They were climbing trees and gathering branches to build a small "fort." Ying was in the garden, picking tomatoes. I was eating a bagel and reading the *Wall Street Journal*. It was odd not to be reading something medical, as I spent little of my spare time doing anything else. As it happened, I came upon an article with the heading, "Survival of the Busiest" and a schematic of a human brain set against a grid of busy circuitry; then, a caption that read, "New Insights Herald a Revolution in Treatment for Stroke, Depression, and other Brain Diseases."

I was no longer entertaining illusions about finding some miracle drug or therapy for my mother. I had decided there were a number of ways to attack the disease of which direct frontal assault through pharmaceuticals was only one. Rehab and therapy were others. The act of study, which I interpreted as an extension of prayer, was yet another (for those of faith), this falling more under the rubric of "healing."

Healing was difficult to prove, yet I convinced myself that such efforts were not futile. How God would even recognize one's efforts at prayer or study I could not begin to fathom. Did He somehow detect increases in metabolism within regions of the brain that correlated with the activity of "study," noting increases in glucose uptake, like a Divine PET scan? Or did He operate a step removed from crude physiology, hovering within our psyches, and able to espy our thoughts; or more subtle than that, before the thought had even formed, at the level of intuition? God did not lend himself to direct analysis. He did not provide pieces of himself for study or electron microscopy or DNA analysis. We could know Him scientifically only through the study of His world, the material world, the world of nature, to glimpse the marks and patterns of intelligence whereby we might then engage Him and grasp His purpose.

The article was fascinating. It was adapted from a book about *neuroplasticity*, an interesting word that referred to the ability of the brain to reform itself based on our experiences: the things we did and thought. The brain, the article said, was dynamic and fluid, not just in infancy and childhood, but throughout life; it allotted 'neural real estate' according to the specific demands placed on it, hence the title of the article "Survival of the Busiest," meaning the busier the brain (or sections of the brain), the more integrated and robust.

I had passed through such concepts in my own recent literature search but usually from the perspective of agents promoting axonal sprouting and new synapses, with reassignment of lost function to other areas. But here the emphasis was on the innate capacity of the brain *itself* to allocate additional territory for performing tasks based on demand: the brain reshaping – or reforming – itself.

I had seen how the brain could tap the powers of the immune system to encourage healing through the medium of neuropeptides and how through such chemical mediators the two systems talked to one another. Here the potential for dialogue went on between the brain and itself, predicated on what it was asked to do. How the brain somehow registered this information and determined that additional neural "assets" were needed seemed esoteric. Perhaps, it fell to Him to fit us out with a brain possessed of such powers of perception and transformation, and of capacities to recreate itself, as if *He* had endowed the brain with near-Divine wisdom to take His place in the event of His absence or withdrawal from human affairs.

The article told of a study involving blind subjects who were proficient Braille readers. They hooked the subjects up so that the part of the brain that processed 'touch' could be measured. The pads of their right index finger (the 'reading' finger) were stimulated. The region of the brain found to respond to the stimulation was much greater in the blind Braille readers than in normals. Similar findings were found when the brain was measured while stimulating the fingers of the left hand of right-handed violinists (the left hand fingers being very active in working the strings of the instrument) when compared with non-violinists.

The research demonstrated that the brain had the ability to re-shape itself in response to specified, repetitive activities. What was also provocative was that purely *mental* drill also produced changes in the brain; in other words, imagined exercise repetitions changed the brain as much as the actual physical performance, implying that *thinking* about doing something worked as well as actually doing it.

I had to laugh. This was truly subversive: a rallying cry for the shiftless and lazy – *thinking* about doing something was as good as *doing* it. Why bother getting out of bed in the morning when imagining it had the same effect: the ranks of the unemployed were destined to explode.

Ying brought me an iced tea. I had to leave soon for the hospital to visit Mom. Would it help if I got her to "think" about moving her left leg or arm? Would she even comply with so outlandish a request? Or would she instead look at me as if I was daft.

I gazed at the woods. The kids were still playing. What was with them? They never worried. I could hear them better than I could see them. They were noisy. The view was beautiful, though, the trees lush and full, the deep, rich green of late summer peaking. Tomorrow was Rosh Hashanah.

I thought about my place in the moral universe, feeling unfit. Yet this was the season for redemption. What were my chances for deliverance and how would I know? Was it a sense of repose, as I sensed now filled my mother? Were prayer and repentance enough to assure myself of a return to God's good graces? Would I improve my chances if I gave up my earthly possessions and renounced all attachments to the world? Where to draw the line? What joys was I entitled to? I hovered between renunciation and repentance, of liberating insight (like the Buddhists), and prayer, worship, and forgiveness (like the Jews).

My mother could not move her left side, yet the therapists continued to exercise those limbs, to inspire the memory of movement even though she was paralyzed and numb. It was a fantasy, yet they persisted. Would they look at me stupidly if I suggested they encourage her to *think* about moving her left side to encourage the brain to reshape itself? The brain was endowed with transformative powers and able to restore itself. There were divine mysteries that were equally inscrutable. I could not know the truth with certainty; I could act only on faith, a faith beyond understanding or reason: to believe in a forgiving Lord, in the powers of the brain, of healing for my mother, of redemption for myself.

When I went to the hospital, I planned to call Cliff from her bedside. He had requested I do so because he wanted to speak to Mom himself. He was no longer angry when we spoke, the resentment and bitterness having drained from him. He wanted to come out again with his two children. He was the only brother planning to visit again. I appreciated this.

When I got there, she was resting in bed. She was sleepy but could be aroused. She looked up and said hello. I smiled and kissed her on the forehead. She seemed relaxed. A nurse stuck her head in the door. "She's much more alert than usual for the morning, Dr. Moss," she said. Mom shrugged, unimpressed. "Where are the kids?" she asked.

"They're busy playing." She seemed disappointed.

"How are you?" I asked. She shrugged but raised her right eyebrow.

"Cliff called this morning. He wants to talk to you. I told him we'd call from your bed." She seemed happy.

"But have him call back; it's more expensive from the hospital," she said. This was typical Mom, always worried about money.

I called Cliff and he called back as my mother requested. We talked briefly. Then I held the phone to her ear. All the usual expressions enlivened her face. She asked him about the kids and work, and if he stopped smoking, which, of course, he hadn't. "You got kids, y'know, Cliff, ya gotta stop," she said. She told him she was fine, she had no idea when she would get out. "I really don't know, Cliff. I don't know what will become of me," she said. The words were spoken with poignancy yet detachment. She told him she was continuing her therapy and making very little progress, again speaking as if reporting on someone else. I listened to her raptly, finding her composure remarkable. She was glad that he called; she missed everyone, and couldn't wait to see them. Cliff must have asked her who had called, because she began listing names: "Yeah, Jack and Larry called. Aunt Annie and Sophie. Pamela, too, and Renee."

I had forgiven my mother a variety of sins, she who had suffered through the years. That she could not forget the wound of her divorce from Dad hurt her most. The careful cultivation of bitterness had become a preoccupation for her, a twisted form of nobility, as if she preserved her honor by continuing to despise him. That she let it interfere with so many other aspects of her life, most of all her own personal development and pursuit of interests, was unfortunate, yet it was self-inflicted.

"You shouldn't bother, Cliff, it'll cost you a lot with the kids," she said. She listened, and then: "Alright, kid, just try to get a cheap flight."

I took the phone. "She sounds OK," Cliff said.

"Yeah, she's OK."

"She doesn't sound depressed."

"I know. Strange, through this whole thing, she's been very calm."

We spoke for a while. He was coming out next week. It would be good to see him.

When I got off the phone, Mom's eyes were closed. I watched her for a while, following her breathing, re-assuring myself that she was alive. This was my new fixation, as if anticipating the next catastrophe.

"Ma," I said, and she stirred. "I'll see you."

"OK, kid," she said and returned to sleep.

Years ago, when I was about seven, my mother took me on a bus ride. Riding the bus as a child was an adventure — the mammoth vehicle pulling in and out of stops, making broad turns, careening down the avenues as people and cars scrambled out of its way. Just getting on the bus was a thrill, the bulky metal monster on wheels with a huge glass face lurching into the bus stop, the immense doors folding in and opening like gills on a fish.

There was a strange glass and metal cage bolted to the floor next to the driver that made raucous, metallic noise as it ate your money. The driver rolled his big black steering wheel, as if he was steering a ship, shutting the doors, releasing the brake, and plunging the behemoth forward into the stream of traffic. The bus made sounds as it moved, gasping and wheezing as it pressed ahead. As you walked back to your seat, you saw the different faces, colors, and worlds that inhabited the bus, like a small transient neighborhood, a cross section of the city brought together for a brief journey.

Mom had placed the thirty cents into the machine that covered our fares, and we lugged our shopping bags to the back. As always, she kept me close by. We found two seats facing the front. I sat next to the window. The bus moved on, picking up more passengers, gradually filling up. My mother grabbed my hand as if to reassure herself that I was safe.

It was a weekend, and the streets were busy with traffic and shoppers. The street vendors were out selling hot dogs, pretzels, and sodas, restaurants and pizzerias were open, and retail shops were bustling. Pedestrians of every stripe clogged the sidewalks, and everyone seemed immersed in their hectic lives. I enjoyed the view through the large window like a movie.

A moment later, the satisfied spell broke and my reverie ended. I heard a voice shouting foul things.

"Damn Jews," I heard the voice say.

I did not believe my ears. I looked around nervously but could not identify the source of the terrifying words.

"Stinking Jews," the voice returned, this time louder.

The whole bus seemed collectively taken aback.

"Jews and niggers!" the voice now declared. "That's all there are in this damn city."

I spotted the origin of the unwanted sounds: a man, sturdy and middle aged, and full of crazed indignation. He was standing up and making menacing gestures. People backed away from him, eyes wide with apprehension. He continued hurling the vicious epithets, "Jews and niggers," now at every turn.

I then heard something even more unexpected: another strong voice, this one feminine, which matched equally the fury pouring from the stranger's mouth. "Who the hell are you?" I heard the voice say. I looked at my mother, who had

*spoken these words, and felt my own mouth drop. Her eyes
were cold and beady, like a Doberman's.*

"Ma, be quiet!" I hissed, terrified.

Her eyes fixed on the man.

*"Who the hell are you!" she repeated fiercely, ignoring
me. I gaped at her, wishing she would be quiet.*

*"What are you, a damn Jew?" the man said as if asking
a routine question.*

*"That's right. I'm a Jew!" my mother shouted, almost
choking with anger.*

*"Ma, be quiet. He's crazy," I said, grabbing her hand.
She pulled away and stood up. She grabbed a bar to steady
herself and walked toward him.*

*"Get out of here," I heard her say venomously as she ap-
proached him.*

He looked at her with contempt.

"Mom, leave him alone," I yelled, crying with fear.

*"Get off the bus, now!" my mother shouted. "You Nazi!"
She uttered this with such rage her face shook.*

*The whole bus closely monitored the event. They were
nervous because they were not sure if the man was dangerous, but also exhilarated by the outrageous spectacle occurring under their noses. Here was a petite Jewish woman,
about five feet, with her young son, confronting some crazed
anti-Semite in the middle of a bus.*

"Stinking Jews," he said again.

*"Get out of here!" my mother hissed again through grit-
ted teeth.*

"You heard da lady, get off da bus," someone else shouted.

*I saw the driver looking at his rearview mirror, wonder-
ing what was going on.*

*My mother kept staring at the man as if she was daring
him, almost hoping, it seemed, he would hit her, so she would
have an excuse to rip his tongue out. "Jews and niggers," I
heard him say, but now just muttering to himself, his force
diminished. He was still angry but deflating quickly. He
seemed to want to strike out at my mother but thought better*

*of it. Recognizing the tide had turned, he moved toward the
rear exit.*

"Get off," another man screamed.

*The man promptly descended the stairs and left the bus
as it came to a stop. He disappeared into the crowds and
streets of the city, a Jew-hating crank properly dispatched
and humiliated.*

*Everyone in the bus seemed to breathe a sigh of relief, as
if we had escaped another Bronx event, a brush with danger
that could have gone badly. People were also gazing at my
mother, the woman who bravely defied the man and effectively threw him off the bus. Some nodded and acknowledged
her admiringly. Several began clapping. Others joined in.
Soon, the applause spread through the crowd like a wave,
the entire bus erupting in cheers and huzzahs. Many stood,
roaring and clapping, as if the sight of this pint-sized woman
standing down a bonafide nut had instilled in them a feeling
of hope and pride.*

*At first, Mom did not know what to do; she seemed em-
barrassed. I took her hand. She smiled and bowed, like a little
girl. Then she waved and tears began to form, which only excited the crowd more. I led her to our seat. We sat down as the
applause continued. Mom held my hand, more relaxed now,
smiling and recognizing the sea of faces around her, nodding
to them as if a monarch. Some stopped by as they were getting off, patting her on the shoulder or gently squeezing her
hand.*

*"Wonderful, just wonderful," an older woman said.
"That was great," another said. "God bless you," said another. Others came by to greet and touch her affectionately as
they passed by, offering salutations.*

*Minutes later, we got off the bus and rushed home with
our groceries for dinner.*

- 30 -

I spoke with the neurologist from Indiana University. He was patient as he listened, answering in a polite, professorial tone. He chuckled when I mentioned the bit about "thinking" your way to health, but confessed to not having read the book or seen the research. "It would be great," he said, but wondered how one would know if a patient actually did the thought drills. I reviewed other items I had encountered: neuropeptides, robot-aided neurorehabilitation, amphetamines, osteogenic protein, clomethiazole, fibroblast growth factor, Vinpocetine (the Italian movie star of a compound), aggressive rehab, and others (the long and monotonous list of dead ends, detours, hunches, and fantasies).

I did not bring up prayer. Only the rehab and therapy seemed to resonate with him: preventing contractures and bed sores, increasing circulation, rekindling the memory of movement and sensation, speech and swallowing: all these, he acknowledged, were the standard benefits of these standard treatments. But with this admission came the realization that there were no wonder drugs or treatments awaiting my efforts that would render some startling recovery. He confirmed what I already knew. He agreed that the traditional methods of improving outcomes were most important and that thrombolytics like TPA were of limited use since so few patients met the criteria. He mentioned the risks of TPA and that the media had made a big splash about "clot busters," but the reality was that they were ineffective for the vast majority of stroke patients, not nearly as helpful as they had been for heart disease.

"But then, the brain is a different sort of muscle than the heart," he said, and he snorted at his little joke.

These excursions into stroke research were no longer helpful to me, and the more I indulged the tendencies to uncover what had not been found, the more dismal it became. The purpose was redemptive now, the research a form of prayer, perhaps a kind of atonement. I recognized them as such. Researching my mother's illness was equal to praying. But my mother had imposed no guilt upon me; it was self-imposed, yet even that was now evolving into something else. I felt myself emerging from a dark, labyrinthine cave.

For some reason, in the midst of the call, I remembered the weeping patient whose husband could no longer string words together, nor understand them, the cognitive functions disrupted. I noticed myself not listening to the professor on the other end. I looked at the clock and then at the ceiling and the fluorescent light that was out. I heard the professor wish me well, as if he was at the end of a long tunnel, saying sorry that he couldn't be more helpful. I thanked him from a great distance and hung up. I realized that research and study had run its course, the phone call a fitting end. Study was no longer redemptive; I would have to find peace in some other way. Perhaps, my mother would help me.

There was little discussion of Dad after Larry's wedding, a happy occasion. No one missed him at the affair, and Mom watched, smiling, as her first son was married. Larry was now out of the house. I saw in it some general portent of the inevitability of change in life, something to fear, overall an unhappy condition.

About a year after the wedding, Mom announced that we were moving. She didn't like the old neighborhood; it had "changed," she said; she wanted us to move to a more "Jewish" neighborhood.

She brought us to see the new apartment on University Avenue. She was proud of the big rooms and the beautiful park in front of the building. There was a view of a reservoir across the street, and the schools were nearby, so we wouldn't have to walk far.

"Do you like it kids?" she asked excitedly. The rent was higher, she said, but worth the $110 a month. There was also a synagogue nearby. None of the brothers wanted to move, to find new friends and go to a new school, but no one said anything because Mom seemed so happy with the decision.

Larry had finished college and had gotten a degree in business. We were proud of him and thought that finishing college was a great achievement. Mom wanted him to become a professor. He opened a factory in the garment industry in lower Manhattan with Uncle Morris instead: a "cutting room," he called it. We went to his house or he visited us in our new apartment. I don't know if he visited Dad anymore, since he wasn't at home, but Jack did. He took the train down to see him. Other than his visits to Dad, Jack was a hermit. He stayed in his room and read. He wrote strange things in his notebook about being the "King." He was having trouble in school.

I was preparing for my Bar Mitzvah and took lessons at the local Temple with Mr. Rosenberg. I have always felt guilty about how everyone, including me, in the class treated him. He had certain characteristics that invited ridicule, first of which was that he stank. This was unfortunate because it became the basis of unending jokes and insults. He often looked to me as the class leader to help maintain order. Sometimes, though, I succumbed to my baser instincts and behaved shamelessly like everyone else.

As I approached my thirteenth birthday, my mother decided that she wanted me to have the Bar Mitzvah at a "Sep-

hardic" (Spanish) temple, the one I was currently enrolled
in being "Ashkenazi" (German). For this, it was necessary
to travel by train to Burnside Avenue. The rabbi there was
an olive skinned, elderly man, slightly balding, and a strict
disciplinarian who made it clear that disobedience would not
be tolerated. He did not like my pronunciation of the Hebrew
word "Torah." He yelled, "To-rah," with the accent at the
end; then muttered something about my general incompetence and poor Jewish upbringing.

"You know what it is to be a Jew?" he asked angrily. I
nodded.

"No, you don't know, but you will learn," and he grabbed
my cheek sharply, pinching it. I winced and wondered how
he would have handled the kids in Mr. Rosenberg's class.

At the Sabbath service, the Rabbi called me for **aliyah**
(going up to the Torah) and my Haftarah reading (a section
from the Prophets). I limped through it with no major gaffes
and received an affirmative nod from the Rabbi. He then
placed his tallis over me and recited a blessing for continued learning and growth in Judaism; he handed me a Siddur
(prayer book) as a gift. I then carried the Torah scrolls around
the synagogue where I received the affections and congratulations of the congregation, most of whom I didn't know. That
I was given the honor of reading from and then carrying the
Torah signified that I had become a **Bar Mitzvah,** literally a
"son of the Law," and therefore ready to assume the religious
responsibilities of an adult Jew.

The Torah scrolls were heavy and at one point I stopped
to adjust them. The Rabbi glared at me. I noticed my mother
holding her breath. Then I continued, and the little bubble
of tension dissolved. After the ceremony, my mother kissed
me and said, "Congratulations, son, today you are a man."
We drove over to the reception at a community room in an
apartment building on Boston Road, all paid for by Larry.
There was music, food, and dancing. All the relatives and
friends were there. Dad didn't come. I got a card from him
with a check.

We adjusted to our new apartment and neighborhood. Jack had dropped out of school and was getting an "equivalency" diploma. Jerry was in the tenth grade at DeWitt Clinton High School and not excelling. I was in the seventh grade at Junior High School 143, in an accelerated program for advanced students (the "SPs") 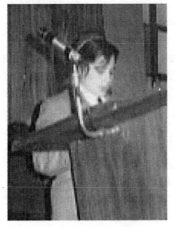 but doing so-so. Cliff was in the fourth grade at PS 86 and getting into fights. Mom rode the train downtown to work as a receptionist. She also did the shopping and cooking. There was a Grand Union right by the train station on Kingsbridge Road. She walked home, about ten blocks, with shopping bags heavy with food. It was tiresome and she was often irritable by the time she arrived. Sometimes Cliff and I met her at the station to help her. Many nights we had TV dinners or lasagna or something else premade that only had to be heated in the oven. Dad had not been around for years, but he reentered our lives a few months later.

The phone rang when I picked it up. It was Larry. He sounded worried. He told me to get Mom. I watched her face, concerned by the tone in Larry's voice. Her reaction to Larry' words over the phone frightened me. It was not an ordinary reaction to bad news, but something much worse, as if she had been slapped sharply in the face. She gasped audibly, and her face grew pale.

"Ohmigod," she said, and almost immediately began to cry. She asked Larry repeatedly, "Are you sure, are you sure?" When Larry hung up, she pressed her head against the wall, moaning as if she had been mortally wounded. When she turned to face her sons, she was trembling. I took

*her hand. She sat on the sofa sobbing, unable to speak. Final-
ly, she told us that Dad was undergoing emergency surgery.*

*Larry drove us to the hospital, where we waited for the
surgeon. He appeared in green scrubs, exhausted, his surgical hat stained with sweat. He told us that Dad had ruptured
a blood vessel in his brain, an "aneurism" he called it. He had
stopped the bleeding but the damage had been done. He was
in a coma and would probably never wake up.*

*"Isn't there something you can do?" Mom asked. He
shook his head grimly. We went to the ICU. Clusters of
drains emptied from Dad's bandaged head and other tubes
escaped from his nose, back, and bladder. He was on a ventilator, slobbering around a breathing tube, his tongue hanging
out, and his eyes half-open and vacant. It was not my father,
I thought, just a carcass, a beating heart and lungs. None of
us stirred from the horrible sight, aghast but mesmerized,
our fixation complete. We were reluctant witnesses to the
spectacle of life sustained artificially, of nature betrayed, of
our once invincible father reduced to drooling pulp.*

*Mom went to the small Jewish temple in the hospital to
pray. She prayed for hours. She stayed there as if doing penance, wondering, perhaps, with a suffocating guilt what her
role may have been in all this; holding vigil for her former
husband, and the father of her children. She knelt, something
I had never seen her do before or since, and she mumbled
frantically, asking God to save my father.*

*Dad died the next day. The entire family, aunts, uncles,
and cousins gathered at our house. Helen told me that Dad
was better off, a notion I rejected vehemently. Not in this
case, she said, holding my hand. My feelings for my father
ran surprisingly deep. I had not seen him in years, but there
were the memories of the early years, of a boisterous, spirited
man who could do no wrong.*

*For Jack, though, it was a catastrophe. He fell onto his
bed as if struck by a sword. "Goodbye, Dad," he cried over
and over. We listened to him weeping, his suffering and torment penetrating the rooms of the house, stirring our own*

sorrow. It went on, a great wound afflicting him and releasing a wide river of anguish. What mix of emotions and guilt may have consumed my mother, I did not know, for she had labored to keep him from his father. She rushed in to console him, her instincts as a mother overwhelming any misgivings she may have had. She rocked him like a baby, weeping with him. Jack did not reject her, for with all her faults, he still loved and needed her.

- 31 -

For Rosh Hashanah, the Jewish New Year, I would spare nothing. I would bring the holiday to her, if such a thing were possible. I informed the nurses of my plans and they prepared her in the lounge. Ying and the kids accompanied me. We brought the proper Jewish symbols of the season: the Kiddush cup, wine, candles, the round Challah bread that I had made, the apples and honey, and the Shofar, the great ram's horn brought from Israel. It was a festive event but also the beginning of the Days of Awe, the season of prayer and repentance that culminated in the Day of Atonement, Yom Kippur, ten days later.

It all seemed fitting, in a way perfectly timed, for I had ended my compulsive research. It was futile, I realized, some game I played to distract myself, although the effort had served its purpose. It was oddly my mother who led the way, she who had already moved past bitterness and remorse. But she was tired tonight, I could see. She did not welcome this. She had always loved the trappings and pageantry of her religion, its majesty and rituals, but her energies were limited and the effort to participate taxing. She seemed content to watch TV and escape into the thoughtless images streaming across the screen.

Ying had readied the candles. I had sliced the apples and arranged them neatly on a plate with a small dish of honey (for a sweet new year). Ying had placed the round Challah (a symbol of the cyclical nature of time, appropriate for the season) on the table with a decorative cover. I poured the grape wine into the Kiddush cup.

"Arielle, say the blessing," I told my five year old. I did this to arouse my mother. And, indeed, after the blessing and the lighting of the candles, Mom cocked her right eyebrow, and beckoned for Arielle to come for a kiss. Noah became jealous; he therefore got to say the blessing for the wine. Mom responded with a smile and a kiss for him, too. Arielle recited the blessing over the bread. We dipped the apples into the honey for a sweet new year. We recited the blessing, "Our God, and God of our people, may this new year be good for us, and sweet."

Despite the joy of the occasion, the beginning of the Jewish New Year, this, the "anniversary" of the creation of the world, Mom remained distracted, stirred only momentarily with displays of Jewish learning by her grandchildren. She still tended to focus on the TV. The television was a wonderful opiate, I thought, and I wound up shutting it off. I wanted her to return to the living and to reacquaint her with normal interaction.

The blowing of the shofar was next. This was done first by Noah, who, at age three, was amazingly gifted. He blew the ram's horn loudly, thus fulfilling the words of Leviticus, ". . . to observe a day of rest, a memorial proclaimed with the blowing of the shofar . . ." He continued playing it like a trumpet, unconcerned with the religious aspects of it. Everyone laughed; Mom smiled. It was funny indeed to see this tiny body making such a racket. Then I recited the traditional greeting to everyone and to my mother, "La shana tovah," I said, "a good year," and with this we formally ushered in the Jewish New Year, the Days of Awe.

I sat down with Mom. She was drifting. "Ma, wake up," I said. She became irritated. "I *am* awake, Rick."

I noticed again her tendency to brush her right hand over her hair as if it were annoying her. "Why do you keep doing that?" I asked. She looked at me resentfully. I stood deliberately to her left to try to get her to turn to the left, her affected side. She tried halfheartedly but with little effect. "Look this way," I said, encouraging her to at least "think" about doing it as the article suggested. She again appeared bitter. I did not want to badger her, but I was also unwilling to abandon her. Since I did not know with certainty that she could not improve, I felt obligated to continue this form of harassment.

The kids amused themselves, playing with one of the nurses, blowing the shofar, coloring Jewish symbols with crayons someone supplied. This was good because I wanted to spend time with Mom without having to entertain them. I remembered her comment, "It's not your fault." At the time, I was uncertain whether she referred to getting overheated or something else. It did not seem the right time to explore its significance either. Mom was in no mood; she was slowly lapsing into her usual stupor, occasionally responding to something the kids might do or say but otherwise apathetic. I clung, however, to the power of the ten days that was upon us, attaching significance to the convergence of events: the High Holidays, her illness, and my failure. It was a time of redemption.

Noah came over with a picture he had drawn of a Jewish star. "Good job, Noah," Mom said. And she raised her right hand, beckoning him for a kiss. She could not turn her head to deliver it, and only the right side of her lips functioned; but she managed to bestow a limp, crooked kiss upon her grandson, after he dutifully placed his head in the precise position for her to do so.

Jerry called the next morning, wondering about his mother, and whether I had made arrangements with

TriStateRehab. I told him that indeed I had and proceeded to review the pros and cons of the plan. TriState was well recognized in the area, highly recommended, and would represent a more aggressive approach to her rehabilitation than she was currently getting. It would however be an hour's drive and visiting would be difficult, perhaps limited to weekends. But it would not go on forever, perhaps a month or so, at which time we could assess her progress.

I was not sure if Mom would have an opinion; perhaps she would prefer to leave it to me, or perhaps she would prefer to do nothing. In her more animated moments, perhaps, she could weigh the option for herself. In any event, an initial evaluation was needed first, and was scheduled for later in the week. Jerry was concerned that Mom wasn't being pressed enough, that left to her own devices she would acquiesce to her miserable status and continue her decline. He argued forcefully that the disease and degree of disability had not unequivocally declared itself and that there was still hope that with dedicated effort another centimeter or so of improvement might be squeezed out. I was happy to hear his concerns, glad that he worried over his mother as I did. His logic was good, his intentions impeccable and, other than his typically annoying tone, I was in full agreement.

At my father's funeral, the casket was open because his second wife was a Christian. When Nono died, we didn't see the body. He was covered in white cloth, like all Jews, rich or poor, and buried the next day. And we couldn't look at him. We could touch him through the covering and put flowers on him or cry against his body like my mother did, but we couldn't see him. My mother said it was a sin to gaze upon the dead, that Jews didn't do that, in respect. So, I'd never seen an open casket before like this one for Dad, and I didn't

*like it: with all the flowers and wreaths and bright lights, and
Dad in his blue suit like a wrapped fish. His forehead was
creased, and he had two deep grooves between his eyebrows
where he frowned. His hands were folded over his chest like
clumps of clay, and his lips were pressed and wrinkled like
leather.*

*I kept waiting for him to say something, to remove the
ugly mask, open his mouth and let out one of those deep
coughs, or just climb out of the casket and tell us it was all
a joke. I thought the real body was somewhere else, and they
put this wax dummy here instead for everyone to cry over.
And what was the story with death anyway? Did you really just lay there all the time without moving or talking?
Did your skin really disappear, leaving dry, dusty bones and
nothing else? It made no sense to me, death. Life was real,
death was not. It had to be a joke.*

*I didn't want to look at him when I first walked in, but
my Uncle Joe took care of that. Uncle Joe was the hunter of
the family, had a closet full of guns, one of those rare Jews
who enjoyed spending weekends sitting in tree stands and
shooting animals, so he knew about death.*

*"Come here, son," he said, and he took my arm and led
me over to the casket. I squirmed slightly, hoping he'd let go,
but Uncle Joe planted me right in front of the casket where
my father could reach out and grab me if he wanted. He put
his hand on my shoulder and said, "Look at your father,
son." I stared at him, at the wonder of death in the flesh.
I expected him to clamber out of the casket and light up a
cigarette or announce that it was all a misunderstanding. I
watched him carefully, looking for signs of life. His hair was
black and wavy, he wore a white shirt and a red tie, knotted up to his throat, and everyone said how good he looked,
which I thought was crazy.*

*There were a lot of people here, too: the whole family from
Mom's side, from Dad's side, and from his second wife's side:
three separate camps gathered here; and people were crying,
so I knew it couldn't be a joke. I realized that this was death;*

that this was how you looked when you died, like a plastic dummy; that you really didn't move or talk or do anything, just lied there like you were dead, that dead meant death, and death was a terrible thing to happen to anyone.

Jerry came over, and Uncle Joe grabbed him, too. We stood together with our hands on the coffin, leaning over the side of it like we were in a theater. Jerry curled his lips in like he was biting them, and he was squirming around, too, but Uncle Joe parked him in his place like me. He hovered over the two of us, making sure we both had a good look. I could see Jerry didn't like the open casket any more than I did. "Ok, boys," Uncle Joe said finally, figuring we had had enough. When we walked away Jerry said, "I didn't know you looked like that when you died."

Uncle Willy was there, and he was mourning his friend "Harry." He talked about the fun they had drinking and going to the races; how they used to go to Gamblers Anonymous, real buddies, and no matter what they said, he and Harry could never turn down a bet. Uncle Saul and Uncle Pucky were there, and Uncle Artie, and the older cousins, Stanley, Bobby, Jerry, Sylvia, and Merilee, and everyone said their farewells, forgiving him all the trouble he had caused now that he was dead. Only Uncle Morris didn't come; he didn't forgive him and didn't want to pay his respects. "No damn good," I heard him once say about Dad. Aunt Libby, his wife, didn't come, or any of his kids. Aunt Sophie, Annie, Ruth, and Rae came and said goodbye.

When my mother came in, everyone made room for her, as if she were the aggrieved, which of course she was although they hadn't been together in years. She walked up to the casket and looked at Dad with moist eyes and called out his name softly, almost as if sharing a private moment with him. "Oh, Harry," she said, through the black veil that covered her face. She placed her hands on his dead hands and wept softly, even beautifully, like a song, bidding farewell, lost in her memories of what they had when they were young, before it fell apart.

Dad's second wife was there, an awkward convergence, but she acknowledged Mom and greeted her respectfully. Something in her manner seemed to give deference to Mom. I was worried that Mom would become angry or emotional when she met her. But they recognized each other through the haze of their misery, and any resentment or jealousy they may have felt seemed consumed by death. They stood together for a moment, mourning the same husband. When the other left, Mom lingered, clinging to these final moments, still in love with the man who had caused her so much pain.

Everyone noticed how much Mom cried, and how much his second wife didn't, and that Mom looked like the one that truly loved Harry. But that didn't matter, no one was competing for the honor, and there was nothing to do about it anyway.

- 32 -

I went up to see Mom in the evening. She was sleeping. I did not wake her. I heard voices behind the drawn curtain that separated Mom from her roommate, a lady in her seventies, who had a knee replacement. She was chatting with her niece, Maureen, a local pharmacist I had gotten to know through work. She was a lively woman, late forties, unmarried, and educated. She called me Rick instead of Dr. Moss, which I did not mind. The aunt had her surgery eight days ago and had been transferred to skilled care. I moved the curtain and said hello.

"Hi, Rick," Maureen answered. I could see her aunt was getting along well, already moving the operated leg, and destined for a full recovery. I felt a vague sense of envy.

"How are you?" I asked.

"Fine," the aunt said. "How's your mother?"

"So-so."

"Is she sleeping now?" Maureen asked, as if wanting to know if she could speak freely. I nodded.

"You know, I love that lady," Maureen said excitedly. I smiled when I heard this. It was typical of her, very direct. "She's an amazing lady; I mean she's so strong. You can tell she's been through a lot. We've gotten to know her. She perks up at night about the time I get in to see my aunt."

I almost laughed, I was so happy to hear this.

"But how's she doing, Rick, with the stroke and everything?"

"It's been slow. She had a bad stroke." I felt the drafts of despair returning. I redirected the conversation to dispel the foul humors.

"So how are you doing?" I said, looking at the aunt.

"Oh, fine, comin' along real good," she said, Hoosier style. "Doc said I ought to be out of here real soon, maybe a week, but I'm doin' fine." And the divergence here was poignant. This lady anticipated a favorable outcome. For my mother, roughly the same age, the well-placed crumb in a vessel within her brain cast a far longer shadow.

"Your mother talks about you all the time," Maureen said. "I mean she really loves you and her boys. She told us there were five of you. Man, you must have driven her nuts. But, oh, how she talks. You're her life, man, what she lives for."

The aunt shifted and Maureen helped her. She then returned to the topic of my mother. "And she loves your kids, Rick, just loves them. She was tellin' us how they were doing the prayers in Hebrew for Rosh Hashanah." This surprised me. I thought Mom had been inattentive. "I know about Jewish people," she continued. "I had Jewish friends when I went to college. Your Mom was showin' us that Jewish star she got from your brother Jerry from Israel. It's special, man."

Maureen had captured the essence of my mother – her children and Judaism. I was thrilled that Mom had felt comfortable to share this with her.

"She grew up in Indiana; had nine kids in her family. Jacob and Rebecca were her parents. She moved to New York in 1931. Man, what a story. And here you are back in Indiana. It's ironic she came here and got sick; as if returning home to Indiana to be with her son." This interpretation of recent events had occurred to me

I heard my mother stirring. I stood up as if to dismiss myself. Maureen looked at me, saying, "You know, Rick, I don't know if you heard, but I was diagnosed with breast cancer." She announced this almost as an afterthought. We spoke further about it, but she was soon encouraging me on to Mom who had awakened. "I love your mother," she said in closing. "She's a saint." So, I thought to myself, are you, and thanked her for her kindness.

I visited my mother with Ying. We came later in the evening based on Maureen's recommendations the night before. Mom responded to our appearance with a degree of verve that I had not seen since the stroke. Her eyes were sharp and lively, her face pink, and a crooked smile adorned her face. She seemed almost to want to get up and greet us formally, as if it were in the realm of possibility.

"Hi, Ying," she said, actually grasping Ying's hand. "You look wonderful."

"Thank you," Ying said, a little taken aback.

"Where are the kids?" Mom asked.

"With the neighbors."

"Everyone fine?"

"Doing fine, Mom," Ying said, smiling.

We sat down. Mom looked at Ying and said, "Thank you for your pendant." This innocent sounding comment was endowed with significance. She was referring to the pendant made of jade and gold that Ying gave her when we returned from Asia. Ying had held it in her hands that first day in Mom's apartment, bowing and then giving it to Mom. "My mother gave it to me many years ago," Ying had told my mother at the time. "It is from China." Mom put it on her necklace, the one with the Jewish star Jerry had given her from Israel, joining the two ancient cultures symbolically on her neck. "Thank you," Mom had said, but somewhat

coldly. Today she had chosen to revisit that little episode by thanking her again, in a different tone, as if to
correct the wrong committed at the time.

"Do you need anything, Mom?" Ying asked.

Mom shook her head.

"We are hoping for your recovery, the children miss
you." And Mom nodded, acknowledging Ying's kind
words.

Mom seemed to study Ying and then asked, "Do
you miss your home, Ying?"

"Yes, I do."

"You should go back for a visit."

"We will. We will take you," Ying said, olive branches now flowing briskly between them.

Mom shrugged, expressing little optimism for such
an event.

"We can hope, Mom," Ying said.

Mom looked at me now and said, "Take her back,
Rick, to her homeland." I nodded, somewhat amused.
We sat together with my mother, the aging Jewish matriarch and the Chinese daughter-in-law, arriving un-
expecedly at a negotiated peace.

*It was TV dinners again. We sat down around the table
and opened the aluminum foil surrounding the rectangular
compartmentalized tins, releasing small puffs of steam. We
cooked them in the oven for 45 minutes, 20 minutes longer
than the instructions said, because I hated the stringy little
veins in the chicken and the extra time made them less slimy.
We had small cups of Coca Cola, valuable stuff, carefully ra-
tioned by my mother. It was chicken with mashed potatoes
and gravy, string beans, and pudding for dessert. The four
of us sat at the table: Mom, Cliff, Jerry, and me. My mother
was still in her work clothes. She was tired and testy. She had
taken the train in the morning down to 42nd street, where*

she worked in the garment district. She came home in the evening after the one-hour train ride, shopped at the Grand Union, and trudged home carrying shopping bags crammed with food, exhausted.

It was quiet around the table, each of us lost in our own little worlds. Cliff was in the eighth grade and taking on attitude fast. He was distant and beginning to assume the totems of the age: long hair, torn dungarees, sandals, beads, and the like. I was in the eleventh grade, also very much enamored of the counterculture and its emblems. Jerry was out of school, out of work, out of mind.

Jerry usually didn't eat with us. He stayed in his room during meals – to avoid Mom and to work off a good head. Mom suspected he was using drugs but had not confronted him. But there was something obviously wrong with him.

I looked up to Jerry. He was a kind of folk hero to me. Selling drugs, stoned all the time. As a young radical, I saw it in a political light, an expression of resistance to the status quo. Jerry had turned me on to hashish when I was fourteen in the same kitchen we were eating in now. Mom was out for the afternoon. He pulled out his stash and lit up. It hit me all at once.

"Good stuff," he said. I started laughing. I didn't know why. All I could do was laugh. And I knew that I liked it.

Mom sat down and looked at her three children. She wondered how our days went. Cliff mumbled something out of the corner of his mouth, barely audible. "Ok, Ma, nothin' special, no problems." She looked at Jerry. His eyes were glazed. I told him before the meal to stay in his room. He thought he was fine and came out for dinner. I had been shielding him from Mom for months: from the drugged stupors, the phone calls, the knocks on the door, the junkies calling out from the street to our third floor window in stoned out, junkie fashion: "Hey, Bubbbaaaaa"(his nickname). And Jerry tossing them little bags of dope from the window. Mom asked me how school was today. Actually, it was one of my official "cut" days when I didn't bother going, riding the bus

to Orchid Beach to hang out instead - but I told her everything was fine. She didn't worry about me so much because
my grades were good. Cliff was another story.

Mom wasn't paying much attention to Jerry, but she
noticed his eyes. She had dipped her fried chicken leg in the
gravy and was nibbling on it. She was tired from the long
day, beset by her own problems and worries. But as weary
as she may have been, she couldn't ignore Jerry's eyes. They
were glazed, yes; but also bloodshot and utterly vacant. At
first, she looked away, confused by what her own eyes were
seeing and refusing to believe them. She took another bite
of chicken, licking one of her fingers. She wiped her hands
with a napkin. She looked again. And something seemed to
register. She blinked and stiffened slightly. Then she stared,
her mouth dropping.

Jerry had smoked, snorted, swallowed, in varying combinations, every illicit drug out there. He might start out
with a little pot or hash, chase it with uppers or downers as
the mood took him, finish with a little coke or LSD. One day
followed the other in an endless stoned continuum. Later,
he turned to heroin. In no time at all, he was shooting up or
"mainlining" regularly. He became a dealer, which paid for
his habit. He was even making some money. It didn't occur
to him that he could get busted or killed. He went to Harlem
to make his "scores." He took a gun and a machete. None of
this bothered him. Then he "dealt" in the neighborhood, top
shelf, best stuff around, with quite a following: Jerry Moss,
king of the junkies!

Jerry began to nod. His eyes slowly crossed. The lips
parted, and a slight drool formed. His head drifted downward. It held just inches above the mashed potatoes and gravy. Then he lifted his head a bit, eyes now closed. Mom's face
tightened. Her eyes, too, formed a kind of glaze.

"Jerry," she hissed through tight lips, the vermillion
barely showing. No response from the hovering head. And
again she hissed, this time with greater intensity, "Jerry!"
And somewhere beneath the dense fog, a glimmer of light

appeared. His head lifted. Then he looked down again and shook his head, little rapid movements back and forth. Small bits of spittle dripped from his mouth. I listened in horror as I heard him repeat the familiar refrain I had heard him say so many times before.

"Messed up," *he said. And then he smiled like a moron.*

"What!" *my mother said, choking on her chicken.*

"Wasted, man," *Jerry said, as if responding to her.*

Mom's eyes widened. Tiny jets of air streamed in and out of her nostrils. Jerry laughed in a demented sort of way, utterly stoned, oblivious to the effect his behavior was having on his mother. "Messed up, man, gooooood stufffff," *he said again, laughing idiotically, definitely catching a good buzz. Then his head drifted downward, inch-by-inch. It descended and finally touched down, nose first, into a pool of brown gravy and partially eaten mashed potatoes. And there the head stayed, the stoned out head of Jerry Moss.*

Mom stood up. She yelled, "What's the matter with you?" *She poked at the dense head with her hand as if touching a dead animal.* "Wake up!" *she screamed. I looked away, almost embarrassed. Jerry, however, didn't move. He must have breathed through his mouth because his nose was submerged in the brown gravy, the liquid spreading over the surface of his face in a grimy layer and onto his hair.*

"Jerry, get up!" *Mom said.* "Do you hear me?" *She was angry, but also worried. I stood up. I didn't know how to console her. What could I say? He'll be OK, Ma; he's just stoned on heroin.*

She shook him. "Get up for chrissakes!" *Jerry lifted his head out of the gravy. He drooled like a lunatic.*

"Crap," *I said, trying to stand him up.*

"He's getting outta this house, ya hear me?"

"Ma, I'll bring him into his room."

"You think I'm letting him stay here?"

"I'll get him some help."

"Help! You idiot. Look at this animal."

"I can help him!"

"Help him? He's gettin' out of here."

"I'll take care of it."

"The hell you will."

Jerry looked up for a moment, the gravy dripping from his face. He looked like he wanted to say something but couldn't form the words. Then he fell back into the gravy.

"Oh God in heaven," Mom said.

Cliff and I brought Jerry to his room and laid him down. Mom stormed in right after us, like a commando, and began pilfering his drawers. Dozens of hard-earned little bags filled with heroin – gone, in the blinking of an eye, flushed down the toilet. Bags of pills, marijuana, and hashish – gone, flushed down the toilet. Uppers, downers, tabs of acid – gone, all of them! She muttered and swore and damned Jerry and me and all of us, all of us god awful hippies, all of us stinkin' drug addicts, all of us dirty, pill-popping maniacs, the whole wretched country gone crazy. She found a big chunk of hash, the size of a rock, and threw it out the window.

"How could you do this to your mother?" She found more drugs under the mattress, inside a vase, in pockets of clothing – a cornucopia of illicit street drugs worth thousands of dollars – gone, never to be used. Needles, syringes, coke spoons, cigarette paper, hash pipes, and other assorted drug paraphernalia – gone before the horrific onslaught.

"May you rot in hell," she screamed. "You degenerates! You animals! You swine!"

I called one of Jerry's friends, a guy named Frenchy, who drove by and picked us up in his station wagon. She cursed and spat as we left. She slammed the door behind us and double locked it.

That night we came back well after the lights in the house were out and Mom was asleep, looking for the chunk of hash she had tossed out the window. Using a flashlight and keeping an eye out for Mom, we nervously hunted down the one thing we could salvage. The streets were silent. It was dark. I looked up and thought I saw Mom staring out the window.

"Oh crap, there's Ma!" We scrambled like rabbits to a row of bushes twenty yards away. We watched the window for fifteen minutes, panting heavily. All clear. We returned to our search. Success! We found the hash in a patch of grass right in front of the house. We slept in Frenchy's car, off the side of the road by the Tappan Zee Bridge, 45 minutes from NYC, getting stoned on good stuff.

- 33 -

"I have to hope that our God is a forgiving God," I told Rabbi Goldstein, closing the door in my office so as not to be disturbed. I had seen my last patient. My desk was a demoralizing mess of papers, charts and notes. The Rabbi had kindly agreed to continue our conversation from a week before. "I will tell you, Rabbi, I am not a Reform Jew ready to dispense with any part of Jewish practice I find inconvenient. But I am also not ready to become Orthodox at this point either."

Yom Kippur was approaching, and I was dirty with guilt. The Christians, I thought, had it easy. They had only to appeal to Jesus. No dietary laws. No restrictions on holidays and the Sabbath. No complicated legal code. No Mitzvoth (commandments). But a Jew! *That* was complex.

"The wish to be with God and ask forgiveness is good. That should never be lost. But the desire alone is not enough. How are you different from anyone else with a wish to experience God? The wish to be with God absent Jewish ritual and practice is not Judaism."

"But to worship without depth is an empty ritual," I said. "What about those of us who are striving? Where do we stand in God's eyes if we are lacking in the specifics but full of devotion?"

"He is ready to receive you," he said.

"The Jewish God is a forgiving God like the Christian God?" I asked.

"Yes. None of us is perfect. The Orthodox Jews are not without blemish because they follow the letter of the law. Even our great prophets wavered. Moses himself faltered. It is essential to Jewish belief that our God is a forgiving God; that we are not redeemed without His help; that we depend on His forgiveness."

"And this comes with repentance?"

"Yes, within the context of Jewish practice. But to live with God is not easy. It is a continuing effort. It is a part of the struggle of being a human being in covenant with God."

"Do we believe that God listens?" I asked.

"Yes, of course. Why do it otherwise?"

"And if God extends his hands to us in forgiveness, what are we to offer back?"

"Truth and the avoidance of sin; to do good; to repair the world; to have faith and courage; to fulfill as best we can the *mitzvoth.*"

"And what is my responsibility at the time of prayer?"

"You must present yourself to Him properly. You must know before Whom you stand. There is a relationship with God. In this relationship, you bring your purity in word and deed, and, as much as possible, good intent."

"There must be some standard to which we are held."

"There is – it is moral and ethical behavior."

"What is sin by our lights?"

"Living falsely. Deceit. Not facing one's lies truthfully."

"And when you realize you have sinned?"

"You must repent."

"And Yom Kippur?"

"It is the culmination of a year's worth of repenting. It is the time when we focus more acutely on it. But repentance is an arduous, ongoing process not limited to a single day."

"But there is the possibility of grace?"

"Yes, there is grace. We are alive; that is grace. We are here talking; that is grace. If you are waiting for the Red Sea to part, it will be a while."

"There are days when I cannot stand before Him," I said.

"You must reconfirm your faith."

"I can call upon Him, as I would my Father?"

"He *is* your Father."

I was miserable. My mother was not doing well. "And so all of us have a chance for redemption?"

"Yes. Judaism gives you this time each year to repent and start anew."

"What about my mother?"

"She is not well?"

"No, and I bear responsibility for her condition." I did not want to mention it, but I could not control myself. "She had a severe stroke that could have been reversed if I had acted promptly."

"It is not proper to belittle yourself."

"But I have failed her."

"Then offer your failings to your Father – and to whomsoever you have wronged."

I received many phone calls about Mom from aunts, uncles, cousins, and, of course, my brothers. There were numerous flowers, get-well cards, and other gifts for her, crowding the bedside table and shelves. It all began to blur, though, particularly with the realization that this story would not have a happy conclusion. In many illnesses, there was a trajectory, an anticipated course and recovery, generally leading to a return to health. And so the get-well wishes and expressions of concern were all based upon a certain expectation of recovery.

It became difficult when one could not anticipate such an outcome. And, after a point, it became a tiresome exercise, in which the same old questions became quite discordant, sometimes even painful; unwanted reminders that the arc here did not lead to restoration but a steady decline toward increasing debility. The time frames, too, were unfriendly, sometimes lasting decades, the victims leading often dislocated, even vegetative existences. I wondered where redemption lay in this context, what *healing* meant now.

I enjoyed my calls from Cliff. The hostility had disappeared. He wanted to know how he could help, if I needed anything. Jack also called, concerned but distant, too overwhelmed with his own affairs to get involved emotionally. Jerry called regularly, business like, expecting rapid turnarounds, wondering why she wasn't better already. And then Larry called.

"It'd be good to see you. Mom would love it," I told him over the phone.

Mom loved all her sons. But was it reciprocated? Were the memories too bitter to overlook? I didn't know. I had forgiven Mom her failings. But I didn't know if the brothers felt as I did. Did they love her unconditionally? The doctrine under which I had operated was that all she had done to hold the family together annulled the wrongs, which I perceived as significant but on balance, trivial. I wished she had developed her talents more; been a better grandmother; pursued interests; traveled; or did anything other than continually wring her hands over what was wrong with the lives of her children. But that paled before the grand effort of the early years. Did the others harbor resentments against her that I did not know of?

"Maybe Helen and I will come up," Larry said.

There seemed to be a dichotomy among the brothers. The two youngest, Cliff and I, were reverential towards Mom, while the older two, Jack and Larry, were much more detached. Jerry was in his own camp, breaking things down in actuarial ways, but generally more emotionally involved than the older two. Were the older ones chastened by bad memories of Mom; of her flawed reactions to the matter of their father? I didn't know.

"I hope so," I said.

The day after Mom threw us out of the house, she was on the phone with Mark Cohen, a nephew and former drug addict, who ran a drug rehabilitation program on the Lower East Side in Manhattan. Mom was frantic. Mark knew a Yoga teacher by the name of Swami Rudrananda who had helped drug addicts in the past. She arranged a meeting. Mom took Jerry and me to meet the Swami, a Kundalini Yoga Master whom, Mark told us, went by the name of Rudi.

We rode the train down from the Bronx and into the bowels of Manhattan, getting off at the 8th Street station with that big brown metal cube balanced on a single point in the middle of Third Avenue. The whole way down, Mom scowled at Jerry, furious at him, yet holding her tongue, realizing that she had to help him.

We walked to Tenth Street, to a store with a sign that said, "Rudi's Oriental Antiques." Standing in the doorway was an overweight man with a massive shaven head and an orange t-shirt. He had a round face, fleshy nostrils, and dark, penetrating eyes. He looked at us and then at Jerry. He didn't smile. He kept staring at Jerry. Jerry averted his eyes at first and then looked back. He shifted. The man was big, like a bear. There was something peculiar about him. He did not bother with formalities.

He told us to come in. We passed two large sculptures of fierce warrior gods from India; then a huge Buddha, exquisitely carved that nearly reached the ceiling. There was an ornate and intricately sculpted metal horse and other oriental statues and paintings and the smell of incense. There was also an otherworldly ambience, somewhat disconcerting yet soothing. I felt giddy. The man told us to sit down. There were others present, tending to him; some were male, also garbed in orange t-shirts with shaven, luminous baldheads like him; there were pretty young girls, too, smiling, offering us cups of tea. Jerry mumbled something like, "Thaaank you, maaan, reaally greeaat, maaan."

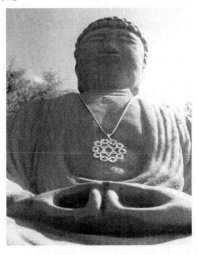

It was baffling, with this big bald guy staring at us, the incense, the bewildering array of oriental images, the other bald guys in orange shirts, and these beautiful nymphs flittering about, offering cups of tea, a kind of new age paradise. My mother seemed skeptical. Jerry was in a stupor. The man sat down on an open chair with a large orange cushion. He crossed his legs in a half-lotus, which surprised me given his girth. He never introduced himself, not even to my mother (which did not please her), but I figured he must be Rudi.

He continued looking at Jerry, never smiling. His manner seemed intended to pierce the dense fog around him, to arouse Jerry from his trance. He took his hand and studied it. He held his other hand on Jerry's head for several moments, closing his eyes as if meditating. He stared at Jerry and said, "You're suspicious, but you'll do." And that was it.

He stood up and beckoned for me. He lifted me up in a magnificent bear hug and kissed me on the side of my head. He smiled for the first time, even laughed. He winked playfully at Mom who remained guarded. Then he kissed her on the cheek and embraced her. He took a deep breath as he held her, meditating briefly with eyes closed, as if somehow absorbing her tensions and fears.

"He'll be OK," he told her.

My mother seemed overwhelmed. "Do you understand his problem?" she asked frantically.

"Of course," he said.

"How will you help him?"

"By awakening him."

"He's a drug addict!" she said desperately.

"He is a self-indulgent child, trapped in his head."

"What will you do?" she said almost pleading.

"I will put him to work. I will break him down. He will confront his ignorance and his tensions and control his mind so he may feel the energy and realize the life force within. The mind is the slayer of the soul. He will learn to control it."

None of this meant very much to my mother who remained confused.

A week later, Jerry was in the "Ashram" in upstate New York, a commune devoted to meditation and spirituality in the Catskill Mountains in the small rustic town of Big Indian. It was a total work scene. Not peace and love. Not bliss and cosmic consciousness, but grueling, physical labor, long hours, seven days a week. No heat or hot water. Cold winters. Jerry lasted four days and was back for a score (heroin). My mother wanted to strangle him.

She said, "Whaddaya doing back so soon?"

He stayed four days with us and returned to the Ashram. He lasted two weeks, then returned to score again.

"What the matter with you?" my mother screamed.

He said he needed some methadone; that he was trying to get off the heroin. He stayed in the house two days and went back.

Two months later, Mom took me up to visit. Jerry's eyes were clear. He didn't drool. He spoke intelligently. He made it through the entire meal without landing in the food. And he worked hard. It was a major turn-around. My mother was thrilled. She went back to thank the man who had saved her son. She began doing "Rudi's Work," as they called it (the meditation practice he taught). She wanted to become a spiritual teacher under Rudi. She was enthralled with the whole "ashram" scene and went up to Big Indian regularly. She found new inspiration that had been missing for years, since her breakup with Dad. Thus began an intense spiritual relationship with Rudi that ended tragically with his death in a plane crash two years later. I was with her when she heard, at Rudi's place in Manhattan where we first met. From this, too, she never recovered.

- 34 -

I went to see Mom that night, purposely arriving late, when all the visitors were gone. I remembered how bright and attentive she had been the last time I had come to see her at night with Ying. It had been a typical day in the office, and I was glad to be done with it, I thought, as I ascended the elevator to my mother's floor: phone calls, complaints, missing operative reports, emergency walk-ins that threw the whole day off, inevitable in such a business. It was a dialectic of sorts, the world of medicine – attending to patients yet moving them in timely fashion so the next patient could be seen – the two efforts at cross purposes, yet both critical to maintaining a successful practice. In the process of finding the middle path, as the Buddhists would say, and balancing the two imponderables, one attained enlightenment. I wondered what constituted enlightenment in the context of my dilemma.

I recalled the conversation with the Rabbi. It was a perspective I had rarely heard in Judaism: the *effort* of Jewish practice, it's demanding, pestering nature; the charge to abide in truth; the requirement to lead an ethical life; the obligation to confront one's lies, deceptions, and sins. How this resonated with me. We sustained ourselves by lies; tarnished and diminished ourselves by lies. Truth, on the other hand, was clear and luminous, universal and eternal, valid and constant, like a law of nature. When one moved away from the truth, distanced oneself from it, and finally lost it, one lost oneself. How to recapture it? How to reclaim oneself? By banishing lies and exchanging them for the passion, strength, and clarity of truth. Only then could one turn to God in good conscious and be redeemed - this was Jewish enlightenment – no less demanding than the Buddhist version. To proceed along such a path was not easy. Yet, I felt I had to.

The elevator door opened. The nurses greeted me. I walked down the long hallway to my mother's room.

There was so much history here, personal and family history, the weight of which overwhelmed me. Whenever I walked into the room with my mother, I felt as if I were entering an old registry with documents and dusty volumes spilling over the tables and shelves.

My mother bridged the gap of two worlds, that of her parents and her children. Her gestures and her expressions, even now with half her face limp, resonated with an old world that had negotiated and eventually made peace with a new one, that had successfully navigated between the ancient ways of a Sephardic community in Macedonia (Monastir), under the dominion of a decaying Ottoman empire (and of her autocratic father), to the streets and culture and freedoms of America. And the admixture had resulted in something quite unique and unexpected: something remorseful and tragic, ill reposed and uncomfortable, yet passionate and vital.

Mom could be stubborn to the point of futility, yet lucent and sincere. She had forged herself under fire, straddling two disconsolate worlds, struggling to maintain composure in an age of utter indulgence that for a time had overtaken her children. She did not seek approval and acceptance in the new era and did not care. She adhered to the ancient verities. She knew from whence she had come and was proud of it, however backward it may have appeared to others.

How I had always loved this menacing little rock in my life. How loyal and steadfast she had been for my brothers and me. When I saw her, she resonated, perhaps inarticulately, this awareness. Her manner, expressions, and voice were infused with it. She was not uncomfortable with who she was. She had wedded me to my family, my people, and my faith, as she herself had been. She had led an imperfect but noble life, untidy but courageous and even inspired. It was hard to do better than that. Jewish enlightenment.

"Hi, Ma, how are you?"

She was reading the local paper, holding it with her right hand, her glasses on. It must seem funny for a New Yorker to read the local paper of a rural town in southern Indiana. The pages recounted the local news of graduations, weddings, deaths, cookouts, fundraisers, high school sports, and the like. She had always enjoyed crossword puzzles but could not do them now. She looked up attentively. The pattern was still in effect. She slept all day and came to life after 8 p.m.

"Hi, Rick, how are you?" she asked with a crooked smile.

I could not say her stroke was my doing. That would be neurotic. The event was purely accidental: the laws of medical science in effect, oblivious and unintentional, as decreed by the Creator, leading inexorably to the accumulation of crud in an artery and a stroke. This was *not* my fault. What *was* my fault was my indolence. How long did I let her sit before responding? Ying had seen it immediately. I dithered aimlessly, a hopeless jerk. There were also the pre-stroke arguments over her personal hygiene, which admittedly had deteriorated, leading to petty squabbles between us. She no longer kept immaculate care of herself as often happened with the elderly. I fought with her to bathe. She took offense. I should have let it go but foolishly confronted her instead.

I did not walk with her as she enjoyed, favoring the kids and their needs, denying her the one simple pleasure we had always enjoyed together. And now she was an invalid. And those moments were gone. I dabbled while she sat there and only when Ying had seen her did the seriousness of the event become evident to me. This was what offended me most, a noxious sore I could not heal. With this my lofty self-assumptions collapsed. I was no longer my own hero but a buffoon.

Then the stupid call to the ER, in which I could not claim with certainty when the stroke started like some klutz, losing the one opportunity I had to save her. She was started on low dose heparin instead of TPA. I did not insist on calling Braun. It was within the three-hour window. It probably would have been safe. The long list of lapses poured forth like acid, unleashing another wave of scalding contempt. If I had acted quickly, the clot may have dissolved. Instead, it progressed, leaving her a cripple. The life and death of one's mother should rest heavily on one's soul. Everywhere I went it was there.

My mother appeared detached from my little drama. She looked at me almost quizzically, and said, "You're an idiot, Rick." I felt as if I had been unmasked, yet I was not offended. I looked at her. She smiled. I smiled back. And then, I'm sure, an amused look must have appeared on my face.

"It wasn't your fault," she said. A magical phrase for me. I had the distinct impression that she knew exactly what she was talking about.

"What do you mean?" I asked.

She did not suffer my foolishness. "I would have had the stroke anyway, regardless of what you did."

I was still mystified but did not bother feigning ignorance: "But I left you," I said. "I didn't help you as I should have."

"Would it have made a difference?"

I remained stunned by her acuity. I did not ask
her to explain it. I hurried past, measuring whether
to divulge the sordid little details. "I left you sitting
in the chair," I said, beginning to unravel before her.
"Ying recognized the problem immediately. I did not.
You could have had medicine that may have helped.
I should have called the neurologist. We could have
used TPA. It could have reversed the stroke." In telling it, I could see I was losing her. She looked away
despairingly.

"What are you doing," she asked, "besides burden-
ing me? You're a big boy, Rick. You know what to do.
I had a stroke and that's it," she said, tears forming.
"You did everything you could."

For the first time since the event began, she looked
at me with deep sadness, as if some unwanted reality
had finally rooted itself within her. My emotions overwhelmed me.

"I disgust myself. I can't live with myself," I said,
breaking down.

"But you can and you will," she said, reaching over
with her right hand to stroke my hair.

"I have nothing but contempt for myself," I said,
holding my head in my hands.

"You have to move on," she said. She looked at me
as she would were I but an erring child, the tears rolling down her cheeks.

"I'm sorry, Mom, for failing you," I cried.

She would not hear of it. She shook her head and
stared at me again. "Enough, Rick," she said. "You did
not cause it. Now stop it!"

I was chastened and felt utterly foolish. I had indulged myself and burdened her. I resolved to control
my emotions. Yet, the moment was significant: the one
whom I had wronged had forgiven me, and after a
complete confession. My relief was profound. I gazed
at the wall behind her, holding back my tears. There

was a wooden figure of Christ on the cross just above her head. How ironic. I doubted she had noticed it since she faced the other way, which was fortunate. On the floor was a pair of slippers, which were useless to her. She was lying down with the head of the bed at 30 degrees. It had been almost three weeks. Yet she looked good. Her lips were pink; hair brushed back, cheeks full. Her eyes were clear and steady, and she smiled. The NG tube was taped to her nose. Somehow, I felt much better.

I told her of my day, the kids, the relatives who had called. I told her about the new Rabbi, our conversations, Yom Kippur coming up. She had enjoyed the Rosh Hashanah ceremony I had brought to her bedside. We spoke about Indiana, her days here as a child. Of her pet dog, "Princee," who died of loneliness when they left it with their cousins after departing for New York in 1931. Indianapolis had changed from when they had lived there: a bigger city now with a thriving downtown, major businesses, professional sports teams, theater, and the arts. Her cousins still lived there, and I had visited them. They still remembered her, called her "Tilly," even though some had not seen her in nearly seventy years. I spoke no further about TPA or delays or failures.

She asked me to pass her bag, the old black leather bag that never left her, even now. She had asked for it right after the stroke, a strange request to me but typical. I had remembered the bag well, all these years, always resting on the stairs of her apartment in Roosevelt Island in New York. It had her cards, phone numbers, cosmetics, pictures, and other essentials. She asked me to open it. She rummaged through it with her right hand and pulled out a silver bracelet, one I had seen before. It had a large sapphire, fine silver mesh spilling over from both sides and a decorative, latticed band, an attractive piece. She held it up and a faint smile crossed her face.

"This was the last gift your father ever gave me," she said almost proudly. I was astonished. "I was not good to him," she continued, "but when he betrayed me I never forgave him. I hurt him in the only way I knew how, which was to keep him from his children. He was a drinker and a carouser. He never had any money. But he loved you kids.

"To this day I'm sorry for what I did. I never talked to you before about this, but it was wrong. You were young, but Larry and Jack were older. They knew their father and loved him. I knew it, too. But I didn't care. I was so bitter. You see how we all do foolish things? And then Larry named his first son after Harry. He was already dead, but I didn't care. I gave Larry hell. 'Do I need a little one running around with *his* name?' I told him. See how foolish I was?"

She continued talking, almost in a monologue. She seemed to enjoy the freedom, yet remained dispassionate and calm. She revealed extraordinary insights and miscues in a long life: about daughters-in-law, children and grandchildren, and, of course, "Harry." She spoke of her failings, her difficulties growing up in a family of nine kids, under Nono, the patriarch, who favored his sons.

Mom had wanted to pursue her education but could not. She was deeply frustrated and had not realized her ambitions or yearnings. She wanted to be a teacher, a professor, a writer, a painter, even a Rabbi. She loved the arts, music, Judaism: none of them pursued. Perhaps, it was inevitable: depression era, large patriarchal family, immigrant parents. Yet her ambitions did not cool or diminish, only sublimated into more palatable forms. But then even as a wife she had failed. And, perhaps, she seemed to imply, as a mother.

I recoiled at the suggestion, protesting loudly. She brushed me aside. She had attached herself to her children with near violent intensity after Dad left, as if to save herself, to salvage some remnant of order and sanity in a chaotic world that had betrayed her. And because of her possessiveness, here, too, she had blundered. I defended her once more. Again she would not hear of it. I thereby enjoined myself not to interfere with her soliloquy; I let her have her full say without comment. I did not fail to notice that even in the telling of her greatest disappointments, she did not seem remorseful. Yet, the admissions were extraordinary, powerful, and, hitherto, unspoken.

When she had finished she held up the bracelet, admiring it. "He was a character, your father. A real con man." She smiled, almost lovingly. "He gave this to me right before he left us." She shook her head, almost laughing to herself. She stared at the bracelet with a look that was both tragic and lovely, still filled with a sense of loss and possibility, forty years after the divorce and then his death, and she now an invalid consigned to her bed. She held it momentarily and then returned it to the bag that she had carried it around in all these years.

She looked at me, her face changed to reflect an inner shifting of sorts. "Get over this, Rick," she said, "I didn't raise you to be a schlemiel."

She had amused herself with this one. She looked at me as if to see how I would take it, and then closed her eyes.

The performance was unprecedented. She had crossed all the forbidden taboos; matters I had always wanted her to discuss, but could never get her to. These were protected realms, cloistered pockets that had festered for years. Now she had exposed them almost casually. I admired her now as I always had, but for completely different reasons. Not for her stubbornness and determination, but for growing up and confronting the wretched little tyrannies that had consumed her, for dispatching her obsessions with boldness and efficiency.

I felt, as I had since the stroke, that I was in the presence of a changed person; one who had, for reasons unknown, undertaken to remove the emotional constraints that had bound her – at her most vulnerable time. It was as if the devastation of her body had created a tiny crack in the rampart of her mind, an opening for her soul to escape.

She aided the process by unloading millstones that had choked her all these years. I cannot say that she was suppressed or muted by her disappointments – her spirit was much too vital for that – only that they had restricted her proper evolution, and she had suffered unnecessarily. She had not fulfilled herself in ways she should have, and for this, I was saddened. But that was over now. Ironically, she was alive and vigorous, her soul flourishing even as it lay tethered to the broken vessel of her body – and, perhaps, because of it.

She opened her eyes and looked at me. She was tired. "Yom Kippur is coming," she said by way of reminding me.

"I know."

"Are you going to fast?"

"Yes."

She nodded and smiled. "Good," and she closed her eyes.

The next evening I appeared at my mother's bedside with two unexpected guests, Arielle and Noah. Arielle had her violin. Noah and I had picked her up at her violin class and then we came to the hospital. It was 8 p.m., late for the kids, but I wanted them to see Mom. The nurses made a fuss about them as we left the elevator. "How big they're getting," said one. Noah and Arielle stood shyly next to me, grasping my hands. Another nurse escorted us to Mom's room.

When we walked in, Mom was resting with eyes closed. She seemed to be sleeping but awakened when she heard us enter. She was not expecting the children and her face brightened. She beckoned with her right hand for them to come. They kissed her. Her face was drawn and somewhat grayish. The nurse placed another pillow under her head.

My intention tonight was to have Arielle play the violin for Mom. Next to hearing her speak Hebrew, I knew of nothing else that excited her as much. She had mastered the difficult piece "Minuet Three" by Bach, that actually sounded good. I asked her to get the violin. She refused. My mother then asked her. She relented. She placed the violin case on my mother's bed and opened it. She hesitated. I encouraged her. She grasped the tiny instrument.

We were not a musical family. There were no musicians even in our extended family. None of our aunts, uncles, or cousins played an instrument. Music had not been a priority. Survival was. Playing a violin, lessons, owning an instrument were not options. The difference in opportunities my children enjoyed in the span of a single generation was remarkable. They, of course, took it for granted.

Arielle tuned the violin. I asked her to play "Minuet Three." I could see how happy my mother was just to see her granddaughter clutching the instrument, let alone actually playing the thing. It was so foreign to her. Did five-year-olds play violins? Arielle rested it on her shoulder, positioned the fingers of her left hand over the strings, and grasped the bow with her right. She arranged her feet and posture. It was a wonderful moment in the history of this otherwise grey hospital room, filled with disease and infirmity.

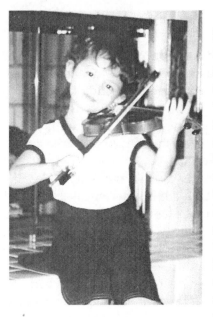

As she began playing, the notes poured forth instantly from the small wooden instrument in soothing waves, filling the room, the corridors, and quarters nearby. She stroked it gracefully with her bow, while the fingers of her left hand rapidly shifted and realigned themselves, the two in a continuous dance, thrusting, countering, and replying to one another, sustaining the magical piece that now filled the spaces with eternal, wondrous sound.

The spectacle of such music emanating from the hands of a five year old was therapy for my mother. She smiled with her eyes closed and moved her head rapturously to the pleasant movement. She inhaled deeply, as if savoring it, in love with the resonances, lost in its harmonies; they, washing over her sumptuously and inducing, it seemed, great joy. There no longer seemed any remorse or regrets.

She went no further than the current note, a fleeting thing as it rapidly blended into the next, rising swiftly and falling, emerging for an instant of time before being overtaken by the next sequence, ephemeral yet everlasting, like a stream. There was only the moment, it seemed, the arrangement of chords, the deftness of tiny fingers, and the euphoric echoes that surrounded her, wrapping her as if a tapestry, transforming her as if an epiphany.

Arielle continued playing her violin, but it was more that she was playing *my mother*. Her roommate opened her curtain. Some of the nurses came in to listen. Mom nodded her approval in grand fashion like a dignitary holding court. Noah, surprisingly, remained still and did nothing to disturb the mood. He seemed content to give Arielle the limelight, as if recognizing that the event was too important to disrupt, too splendid to mingle with petty jealousies.

Arielle finished the piece and played several more at my urging. She did not resist, as would normally have been her tact, sensing somehow that performing was a wonderful offering to her Nona, an exquisite gift too sublime to abort in the midst of such heightened pleasure. She performed for nearly twenty minutes, her small audience spellbound and rapt, and her grandmother ecstatic.

When she finished, she put her violin back in the case. Several of the onlookers applauded. Then the rest joined in, the nurses, aides, and Mom's roommate all smiling admiringly at the small maestro. I beamed proudly at her. She smiled shyly. Mom beckoned and she kissed her and then Noah.

"It was beautiful, Arielle, so beautiful," she said. The little crowd broke up. We stayed a little longer and then left.

I had taken Friday afternoon off to spend it with Mom. It was the day before she had the stroke; a few days after she had arrived from New York.

It was a warm day and the azure sky was lucid and pure with only an occasional cloud buffeting about. The beauty of the day was rich and sensuous, almost a presence you could feel as much as see.

I waited for Mom in my backyard. I looked around and listened, admiring the day. The sun hung in the center of

*the sky like a medallion, the world around us dressed in its
radiant light. Great oak trees pressed against the blue canopy
above. Tall grasses swayed. Cardinals and blue jays chirped.
Butterflies fluttered. A gentle breeze caressed the leaves and
blossoms with a whisper. I studied the crowded woods filled
with birdsong and crickets. I thought I glimpsed the hand of
God. Was it the same amazing God about Whom Mom had
read to me when I was a child?*

*I sensed Him indulging the spectacle of His creation,
wondering, perhaps, if he had been too lavish. Or, perhaps,
reflecting on the laws he founded, the principles that governed time and space, the movement of the heavens that had
evolved into – this. Had he erred in his original formula-
tions? Should he have altered slightly the wave function of
light, adjusted the chemistry that joined atoms into molecules, changed the affinities between the planets and stars, or
was everything . . . perfect?*

*I sensed joy resonating from the earth today, His joy. The
joy of the great God about Whom Mom had spoken; from the
forests and parched meadows, the dusty dirt, and the corn-
fields. A joy that lifted from the earth like a hymn, a primor-
dial chant endowed with creative force. As if the Eternal One
was rejoicing and pouring Himself into every creature and
thing, into the earth itself, drawing us upward, raising us in
ecstasy, to meet Him and praise Him, Creator and created, in
perpetual tandem, in eternity.*

*Yes, there was order in the universe, Divine order. The
day itself proclaimed it. Absolute order reigned and everything was, indeed, perfect. You could glimpse its majesty,
sense its hidden structure, and glean its cryptic design in
the symmetries of nature, in the balanced cadences of the
seasons and the day. The oceans and rivers, sky and wind,
moved according to His dictates. The planets and moons,
sun and stars, sang praises to His glory as they plied their
ancient paths, He whose immutable edicts fixed them in the
heavens and set them on their orbits. There was Intelligence
that crafted the infinite tapestry, Divine Hands that guided*

the movements of atoms and galaxies, and all the riotous ca-
cophony within.

It was, as I would say, my mother's kind of day.

It was also a perfect day for a motorcycle ride.

My Honda Magna and its 700 cc 4 cylinder 4 stroke,
had a carrying capacity of 370 pounds, which meant it could
easily handle my mother and me. The main problem was getting her on it.

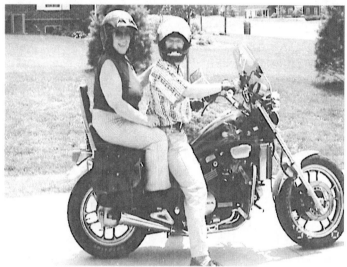

"OK, Mom, get your leg up."

"Oh, God, I'm not as limber as I used to be," she said.

"Here, bend your knee a little."

"I can't get over it, Rick."

"You're almost there."

She grunted and cursed and finally lifted her left leg over
the seat.

"Good, now grab my arm and shift. That's it." She
strained but finally maneuvered herself into position.

"Ready?"

"Uh huh."

I felt nervous at first, riding my seventy-eight-year-old
mother on a motorcycle. If something happened, I would feel
terrible and look like an idiot. "Whut's da matta wit' choo

takin' Ma on a motorcycle, you schmuck," I heard my brothers say in my head.

But then I shifted into second and third gear and settled down.

We drove through town, quite the spectacle for the small hamlet of Jasper, not accustomed to such oddities. We stopped by a clothing store on the square, where the owner was having an outdoor sale.

"Hi, Dr. Moss, how are you?"

"This is my mother from New York."

"A pleasure, Mrs. Moss. Enjoy the ride."

We drove around town, then south on the main road, a few more turns, and then on to an old county road. The sub developments and factories gave way to the burgeoning fields of corn at the height of their season. I turned to my mother.

"You OK, Ma?" And I could see her smiling in the rear view mirror.

The tall rows of corn flew by like a blur and the landscape of southern Indiana in late summer erupted before us: golden meadows of wheat, undulating hillsides, and emerald savannahs dotted by brown and white cows chewing lazily. Silos and barns rose from the dry dirt. Brackish ponds sparkled in the sunlight. Limestone mounds adorned the rich soil like jewelry. The sun passed over us with warm hands today, anointing us, the copper earth, and the speckled patchwork of soy and corn. We plunged through the dense air, mother and son, on a hot metal horse, oblivious and euphoric.

"It's beautiful, huh, Ma."

"Yes," she said with excitement.

"Good ole Indiana."

It was a glorious day, a perfect day, a day beyond imagining.

"It's Jack's birthday," Mom said.

"That's right, September 4, I almost forgot."

We continued on our way, enjoying the green path, the red clay, the pregnant earth, the sultry sky endowed with grace and magic.

- 35 -

Lord, what is man that Thou takest knowledge of him?
Man is like a breath; his days are as a passing shadow.
You sweep him away; he is like a dream.

A psalm of David (144)

My mother died the day after her granddaughter
Arielle had brought her to such heights of joy with her
music. I did not expect it, nor was I prepared. Perhaps,
in retrospect, I should have been. But I could never
have been prepared for this. I was destined to suffer
this, unable to see the emerging patterns, the poetic
symmetries, its inevitability.

It was a Friday, a lovely day, September 25, the
Sabbath, "*Shabbat Shuvah,*" a special Sabbath, the Sab-
bath that fell between Rosh Hashanah and Yom Kip-
pur, when the words of the prophet Hosea were heard.
"Shuvah Yisra-el," he said, "Return O Israel, to thy
God; for thou hast fallen by thine iniquity."

I received the call from Regan in the town of Paoli,
where I held a clinic once a week. He told me of some
calamity that had befallen her, the nature of which was
uncertain. A heart attack, a major stroke, a pulmonary
embolus, he could not say. She was still alive, but barely so. He asked me what I wanted to do. It was a hid-
eous question, for it thrust the terrible reality upon me.
He wanted to know whether to continue advanced life

support or not, and whether to resuscitate her in the event she arrested.

I was numb but answered. "Keep her alive," I heard myself say.

"Full code?" a voice on the phone pressed.

"Yes. I'm leaving now."

I cancelled the clinic. I grabbed my bag. "My mother's dying," I told the receptionist. The words were profanities. I wanted to spit. I saw the receptionist's face. She was full of compassion.

I was unready for the catastrophe; unready for these wretched crumbs, these rotten things that had wrecked my mother's life: plaques and clots: disgusting things. I despised them all. Disease and death. Strokes. They were abominations.

I got in my car. I wept like the baby my mother had raised.

When I arrived in Jasper, I did not go immediately to the hospital. I hoped the delay would not cost me. But I knew I would need my prayer book. This was already a cruel admission. And I needed a shirt - a black shirt and a scissor to cut *keriah*, the ritual tearing of one's garment upon hearing of a death. And then I drove to the hospital. Ying was there. She comforted me. It was room 338, the ICU.

It was an appalling sight – the tube down her throat, taped to her mouth, cutting into her flesh; the ventilator; the lines and drips; the cursed monitor with its luminous squiggles and numbers; her vital signs in disarray. The nurse regulated the medicines that now sustained her. I looked at the spectacle, for me a nightmare, offensive and caustic, like acid.

The nurse stayed in the room, fastidiously watching vital signs and adjusting drips, pestering me with her presence. I wanted to be alone with my mother, to talk with her, to comfort her, she who had suffered so. I saw her small hands, the delicate little hands that had held me. I looked at her face, her lips, and all the familiar features that would soon be gone. Her eyes were partially opened but not seeing, and I cried at her unseeing eyes, the blank eyes that had once looked at me with such affection. I held her little hands.

"Momma," I cried, like a little boy, "I'm with you. Do you hear me, Ma?" And I was happy that at least she was alive, that I could be with her before she died. I was uncertain of her brain activity, of her ability to perceive anything, but it didn't matter. I cared only that her heart was still beating, the blood still flowing through her veins, that I was with her, and she was alive. I ignored the nurse who continued her fidgeting. And then she said something I liked. She said, "Her blood pressure has come up since you got here, Dr. Moss."

And shortly after that she arrested. And with that came the horrendous effort; nurses pounding on her chest; aides rushing about; pharmacists drawing up medicines. Regan appeared. He opened the line; wheeled in a pacer; arranged paddles; shocked her; thumped her chest; called for adrenalin. There was more pounding; more shocking; more flailing, but no rhythm.

I could not stand the violence, yet did not put an end to it. Regan increased the voltage and shocked her again. She flailed horribly, her arms and legs flying off the bed, and Regan looked at me as if to ask why I was putting her through this, that she was dead already, and that our efforts were futile. But then a rhythm suddenly appeared: a puny, stunted thing, nothing that would sustain her, but at least not flat. Regan looked at me plaintively, as if to say there was nothing more he could do. I perceived it as a gift, and said, "Enough."

And with this, the frenzied activity to keep her alive ended. In its place was a penetrating stillness - the stillness of approaching death. The nurses moved the carts and other paraphernalia from the room, arranged her blankets, and tidied up the room. And I was left alone with my mother and her heart beat. I put my yarmulke on and held her hand. I wept as I felt her fragile pulse sink into oblivion. I looked at her face and recited on her behalf the deathbed confessional she could not say herself:

"I acknowledge before you, O Lord my God and God of my ancestors that my life and death are in your hands. May my death atone for whatever sins I have committed before You. In Your mercy, grant me the goodness that awaits the righteous and bring me to eternal life. May you guard my loved ones to whom my soul is joined. Into Your hands I commend my spirit, for You will redeem me, eternally faithful God."

The flat line returned. And she died. At 6:10 p.m., September 25, 1998, on Shabbat Shuvah, the Sabbath of Return.

I closed her eyes. But I did not cover her face. I recited the Shema: "Hear, O, Israel, the Lord is God, the Lord is One." And as I spoke the words, the tears fell from my eyes. And then I cut *keriah,* the ritual tear made in one's garment, my black shirt, next to the heart, a tear that will never be mended. "Praised art Thou, O Lord, the true judge," I said.

And where chaos and violence had consumed the last minutes of my mother's life, there was now silence. And in the vastness of that silence, I felt something splitting within me, as if some terrible knife were at work, carving wickedly and feverishly in the most horrid of places. I heard my mute howls echoing insanely amidst the entrails and blood. I was falling. My soul vanished. My mind cleaved, my thought processes splintered and useless. I heard a dull, noxious whine: the sound of my torment and disorder. I stared at her lifeless body and caressed her face and hands. I held the Jewish star around her neck, my tears mingling with the beautiful silver from Israel.

"Momma," I cried out like a child, "Momma," I said over and over. I could not bear the separation, the rupture, the dislocation. She who had given me life could not be gone! The finality of death wrapped around me like a dense cocoon; too absolute and immutable to accept, the abandonment and pain too intolerable. Her loss trapped me in its immensity, pinning me like an insect. I struggled horribly against it. I watched my breath escape, the water rushing in around me, into my nostrils and lungs, pressing my flesh, twisting me, snapping my bones. A terrible curtain had fallen that divided us. I could not reach her. I flailed helplessly against the obscure wall. I cursed at the darkness. I was desolate and barren, my grief overwhelming me. Where was she beyond the shadows and the darkness?

I had a vision of a younger mother and a park. It was the old park across the street in the Bronx, when I was three. It was a beautiful day. Her hair was full and black, her eyes gleaming. She held my hand as we walked among the trees, covered by the canopy of leaves above. The sun was setting, a wondrous sunset with orange and purple lines streaking the sky and coloring the clouds.

She smiled, eyes closed. Peace and redemption were upon her; joy emanated from her. She told me again that she wanted to paint the sky. She laughed and smiled at her little boy. She was ecstatic with love. And I believed her and adored her, my mother of passion, who taught me to love the sky and the heavens.

I sat with her for six hours, the two of us alone in the room as we awaited my brothers, all of who were coming. It was the Sabbath, and together we welcomed the Sabbath, the day of rest, on this, the Sabbath of Return. And the tears ran from my eyes and onto the prayer book as I recited the Sabbath blessings:

Come, let us sing praises unto the Lord,
Let us sing for joy to the Rock of our salvation.
Let us come before his presence with thanksgiving,
With songs let us sing to Him in joy.

Psalm 95

I read to her and did not stop. I wept for all the Sabbaths we had enjoyed together and for this final one. I read of a woman who had lost a child and went to a teacher for solace. She cried terribly for the pain. The teacher listened patiently and said, "I cannot wipe away your tears. I can only show you how to make them holy with prayer." And I so liked this: to make the pain and the tears holy with prayer. I continued reading to my mother, as she rested, her struggles now over.

Out of the depths I call to You, Eternal One.
O God, hearken to my voice.

Psalm 130:1

. . . Our years come to an end like a sigh.
They are soon gone, and we fly away.
Let Your favor, Eternal One, our God, be with us,
and may our work have lasting value.
May the work of our hands be enduring.

Psalm 90

I was so taken by the final line of that psalm, "May the work of our hands be enduring," for here I saw meaning in my life, for I identified myself as the work of my mother's hands; that my work and all that I had done had been her work; that all that I would ever do was her work; that through her children, who were *her* work, she would endure; in this way she would live forever. And I promised her aloud that all good that had come or would come from me would be in her name, in her honor, in her memory.

Your sun will not go down again,
your moon will not depart;
for the Eternal One will be your light forever,
and your days of mourning ended.

Isaiah 60

I read for six hours. A penance, a duty, a love. I did not stop reading. I stood vigil and confirmed the faith she had loved so much. I promised her through the tears of my love for her. And when my brothers came at midnight, I told them of all that had happened; of the sanctity of sorrow raised up and made holy; that we were the work of Mom's hands; that her work shall endure through us; that we should endeavor to do well to sanctify her life.

I spoke as if possessed, mouthing words that originated from elsewhere, perhaps incoherently. They humored me, wondering if I were touched. They stood at her bedside, stroking her, not fully believing their senses, weeping quietly. I realized how private sadness was, how fortunate I was to have had six hours alone with her in death.

When they were done, we covered her face with a sheet. We kissed her through the sheet and said farewell. Then we left our mother. Jerry had already made arrangements. She would be buried in New York in the family plot, next to her brothers and sisters, who had already died or would die, where we could visit them all together.

-36-

EPILOGUE

My soul thirsts, yea, it yearns for the courts of the Lord;
My soul and body sing joyously unto the living God.

Psalm 84

I recited Kaddish for a year: the Mourner's Kaddish, the prayer that said nothing of the deceased but praised only God as if to emphasize that even under the greatest duress, the most painful loss, our devotion to God was not diminished – and to help redeem her soul. Not in a minyan (a quorum of ten male Jews), mind you, as required by orthodoxy, but by myself: in my office, at home, in the woods.

I was not truly among the living for a year. I experienced no joy, did not laugh or smile, remained numb: the world made colorless, bleak, and flat. It was not depression, but more as if I were a ghost dwelling amidst the shadows, seeking refuge from light, in a barren landscape, in a desolate field, in an arid desert. I wandered hopelessly like a wraith, empty and void, without form or structure, more phantom than real. I was crippled and unfit, yet the darkness allowed me to listen for her voice. My brothers recovered quickly. I did not. People told me to cheer up. I looked at them as if they were daft. Why should I cheer up when my mother was dead?

I spoke regularly to her. I felt her presence most outside, with the sky and the stars she had always loved, in nature. I spoke at the funeral, as did my brothers. My voice was weak, yet sustained itself, a low deathlike rasp to match the occasion. I told of my "beautiful mother," of her final weeks of life, of her return to her ancestral home of Indiana in the splendid month of September, to die. We sat Shiva at Cliff's house, cut short by Yom Kippur.

I returned to New York to help my brothers undo her apartment, this, perhaps, the cruelest day of all. All of her possessions to be confronted and dispersed: the photos, letters, knick-knacks, mementos, furniture, and clothes: things that went back decades: her wedding pictures, pictures of her kids and grandkids, her brothers and sisters, of family occasions. Her kitchen utensils: the old chestnut warmer from Crotona Park, the special pots for making Sephardic dishes – stuffed peppers, spinach meatballs, *fijones*. The trays she used for the *borekus* and *pastel*.

There were her paintings. Letters she wrote as a young girl. Postcards we had written from camp. Plates and silverware, lamps, chairs, jewelry, clocks, vases, books, menorahs, yarmulkes, candle holders, mezuzahs, the sewing machine and scissors, the metal box where she kept her needles and thread to sew our clothes: all of her earthly belongings, each little item resonant with memory and emotion. And we undid them all. Like vandals. Each taking what he wanted, donating some of it to thrift shops, and discarding the rest like so much rubbish, to be scattered about the earth, a form of dismemberment.

I harbored some irrational notion that she was alive through her things, and with this final dispersal, her death was now complete; that in undoing her apartment, we had violated her and contributed to her death. I felt contempt for the vulgarity of it, this final pillaging and violence against her. I apologized to her for the indignity.

I prayed and spoke to her in each of the vacated rooms. Her earthly possessions gone. Her home reduced to chipped walls, dusty floors, and empty closets: the stark, barren spaces where a life had been lived. I knelt and kissed the walls she had lived within. I said farewell to her, looking for her now within myself, listening for her small, still voice. I thanked her for giving me life, for sustaining my brothers and me, for the countless sacrifices she had made. My brothers knew nothing of Jewish practice, but I prevailed upon them to hobble through a brief prayer service and recitation of the Kaddish, to make holy this unholy event.

I spoke with the Rabbi and told him of my despair. The crushing waves of grief that I could not quell. I did not know if it was pathologic to dwell on it as I did. But I was not ready to get "over" it. The pain would move from me in its time. Grief and sorrow were welcome in me as honored guests.

The Rabbi, to his credit, agreed. He offered the usual bromides about "carving" out time for grief. Much of what he said was insightful. "The sorrow," he said, "will help you get to the other side. It will transform and redeem you."

I listened.

"Pain is a knife," he said, "that can cut through the layers and get to the truth. The pain will lessen. It is an opportunity to understand yourself, to remember your mother, and to thank her."

"But what do I do with the pain?" I asked.

"You can burn it up. Through prayer, through the creative process. Since you like writing, maybe you can write a book."

"I cannot bear it."

"Ask God to help you."

"I have regrets."

"She absolved you."

I nodded.

"You loved her," he said softly.

"I know."

"You did everything you could," he said.

"But I did not heal her."

"She was healed. God healed her. She was peaceful. She was calm. She was whole and complete before her death. She came out to be with her son whom she loved, her son the physician, in the land where she was born, away from New York and her lonely apartment to die. She knew. God led her here. Her death was the final healing."

A month later, Maureen, the niece of my mother's roommate in the hospital, came in to see me in my office. It was busy, but I was happy to see her. I did not know why she had come, but I thought it might be about Mom. She told me she was with her the final night when Arielle had played her violin. She had seen her right after the kids and I had left.

"Your mother was something that night, Rick," she said. "She was ecstatic. She kept talking about Arielle, and her recital. She repeated Arielle's name over and over. She said it with such passion. It was so rich. Like music. It rolled out of her mouth like a song. She was happy, Rick. Her eyes were gleaming. She was full of love. She showed us her Jewish star. She kept talking about you and your daughter. I wanted you to know she was happy."

I will turn their mourning into joy,
I will comfort them, and give them gladness for sorrow.
Jeremiah 31

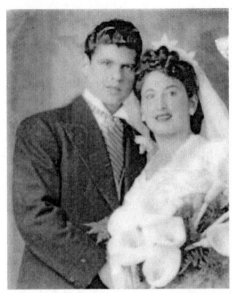

Harry and Matilda

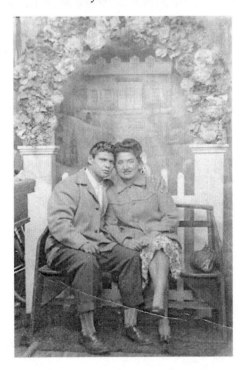

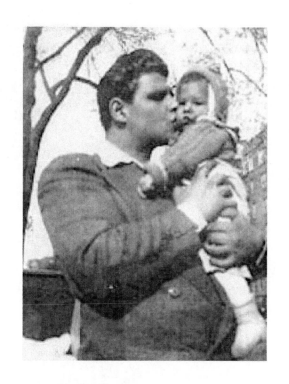

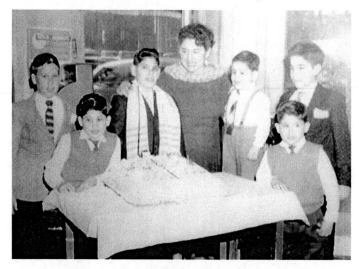

Larry's Bar Mitzvah

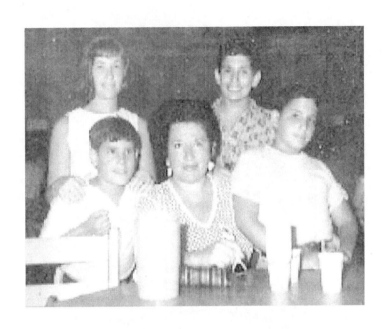

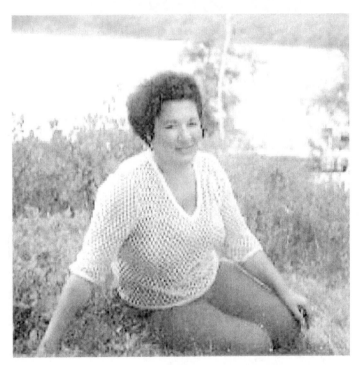

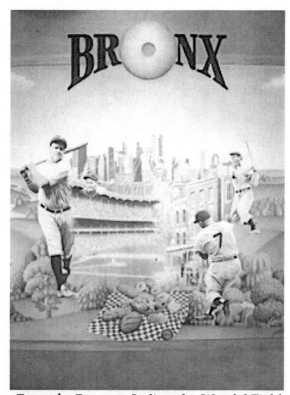

From the Bronx to Indiana by Wendel Field

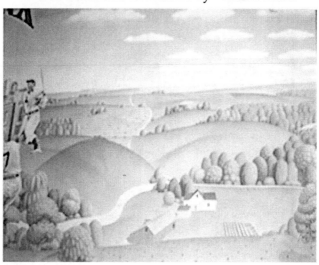

Paintings by Matilda

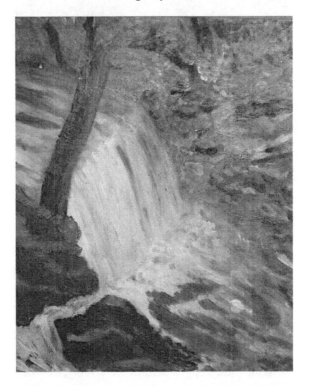

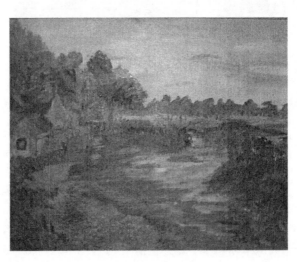

The Author and Family

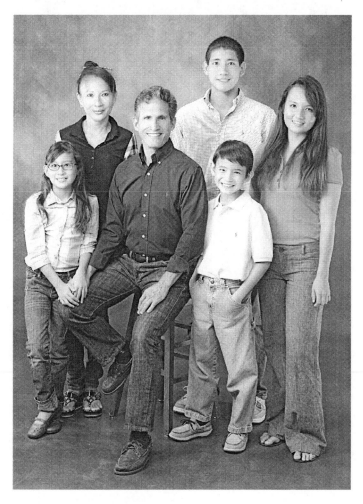

To my Mother, of blessed memory

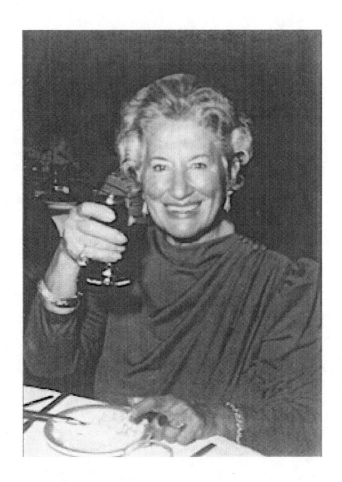

ABOUT THE AUTHOR

Dr. Moss is an Otolaryngologist-Head and Neck Surgeon in private practice in the southern Indiana town of Jasper since 1991 where he resides with his wife and four children. A native of New York City, he earned his undergraduate degree at Indiana University, in Bloomington and completed his Doctor of Medicine at the I.U. School of Medicine in Indianapolis in 1981.

Following a four-year residency in Otolaryngology-Head and Neck Surgery at the New York Eye and Ear Infirmary, Dr. Moss was board certified in 1986. He completed a fellowship in Facial Plastics and Reconstructive Surgery at the University of California in 1987.

Between 1987 and 1990, Dr. Moss traveled extensively through Asia, serving voluntarily as visiting surgeon at medical centers in Thailand, Nepal, India, and Bangladesh. Dr. Moss continues to work overseas. His most recent such journeys were to Myanmar (Burma) in 2004, Thailand in 2009, and Uzbekistan in 2010.

He is an adjunct Assistant Clinical Professor of Otolaryngology at Indiana University. He has published professional articles in prominent Otolaryngology journals and has been a fellow of the American Academy of Otolaryngology–Head and Neck Surgery.

Along the way, Dr. Moss found time to own and manage a bagel shop ("Bronx Bagel") and an Italian restaurant ("Simply Pasta"), teach Yoga and develop a Yoga TV program, "Yoga For Health."

Dr. Moss has always loved writing, at first wanting to become a journalist before deciding on medicine. He wrote essays and helped create an "underground" newspaper, *The Isabella*, while a student at Columbus High School in the Bronx. He wrote essays, poetry, and travel stories while a college and medical student for local and regional papers in Bloomington (*Primo Times*) and Indianapolis (*Indianapolis Star*). He wrote a book based on his travels through Asia as a surgeon, *The Cutting Edge*.

While overseas, Dr. Moss wrote frequent columns, travel pieces, and human-interest stories for the *Bangladesh Observer*, the *Bangkok Post*, and the *Nation* (Bangkok). Dr. Moss has written several magazine pieces.

He continues to write newspaper columns and feature stories for a variety of local and regional newspapers in Indiana. The articles cover a range of topics including religion, travel, and politics. He maintains a blog and website, exodusmd.com.

About the Book Cover by Artist Wendel Field

Years ago, Wendel Field agreed to paint a portrait of my mother using one of my favorite photos of her. The original plan expanded to become a detailed study of the family tree, centered on my mother but extending upwards to include her five sons and three of my four children, her siblings and their spouses, and her parents and grandparents below. The canvas includes the trajectory of one branch of the Jewish people of which we are a part, the Sephardim or Jews of Spanish descent. It begins at the bottom with iconic biblical figures (Moses and Abraham), an image taken from the Alhambra in Spain and a silhouette of the Blue Mosque in (Istanbul) Turkey, where many Sephardim (including my ancestors) fled after their "expulsion" from Spain in 1492. Monument Circle in Indianapolis symbolizes the city where my mother's parents emigrated; images of the Bronx, where my mother's family moved in 1931, and where my four brothers and I were born and raised.

There is a menorah in the background, a man blowing the shofar, a dreidel, lulav, Passover Seder plate, Sabbath table, Torah, and other religious objects. It is a compressed but poignant portrayal of the life of my mother, our family, and large swaths of the Jewish people.

Wendel granted us permission to use his painting(s) in this book. (For more information about Wendel, visit his website at www.wendel.us).

Wendel Field's Artwork on Page 361

This piece by Wendel Field is an epic work painted for the Bronx Bagel, a bagel shop/restaurant I owned years ago. It spanned nearly an entire wall, some twenty by seven feet in dimension. It merged the disparate worlds of New York City (emphasizing the Bronx, where I am from) and southern Indiana (where I have lived most of my adult life). As you scan the painting from one end to the other, you move gently from the soothing, pastoral countryside of rural Indiana, to the charged, turbulent world of New York, and back again, seamlessly, to Indiana's rolling hills.

The painting inadvertently (as it was completed well before the book was conceived) captures elements within the story, and brings together, like the book, the two antipodal worlds of southern Indiana and the Bronx.

367

BIBLIOGRAPHY/RESOURCES/ARTICLES

Morgenstern, LB. What Have We Learned From Clinical Neuroprotective Trials? Neurology 2001; 57 (suppl 2) S45-S47

Krebs HI, Hogan N, Aisen ML, Volpe BT. Robot Aided Neurorehabilitation. IEEE: Transactions On Rehabilitation Engineering, Vol 6, No. 1 March 1998; 75-87

Adler J. Strokes. Newsweek, March 8, 2004; 43-48.

Carmichael M. How A Brain. Newsweek, March 8, 2004; 49

Geldmacher DS. Enhancing Recovery From Ischemic Stroke. Neurosurgery Clinics of North America, vol 8, No. 2 April 1997; 245-251

Gladstone DJ, Black SE. Enhancing Recovery After Stroke With Noradrenergic Pharmacotherapy: A New Frontier? Can J. Neurol. Sci, Vol 27, No. 2 May 2000; 97-105

Ren JM, Kaplan PL, Charette MF, Speller H, Finkelstein SP. Time Window of Intracisternal Oseogenic Protein-1 in Enhancing Functional Recovery After Stroke. J Neuropharmacology, 39, 2000; 860-865

Lyden P, Shuaib A, Ng K, Levin K, Atkinson RP, Rajput A, Wechsler L, Ashwood T, Claesson L, Odergren T, Salazar-Grueso E. Clomethizole Acute Stroke Study in Ischemic Stroke (CLASS-1): Final Results (with editorial comment by Hankey GJ). Stroke. Vol 33(1), January 2002; 122-129

Krause GS, White BC. Cerebral Ischemia. Study Guide in Emergency Medicine, Judith Tintinalli (et al), Section 2 Resuscitative Problems and Techniques; 65-67

Be Stroke Smart, National Stroke Association, Volume 15, Special Prevention Issue 1998

Caprie Steering Committee. A Randomized, Blinded, Trial of Clopidogrel versus Aspirin in Patients at Risk of Ischaemic Events (CAPRIE), Lancet, 1996, Vol 348 No. 9038;1329-1339

Johnson K., Intracranial Stenting Shows Promise. Medical Tribune Neurology Edition, March 1999, Vol 2, No 2

National Institute of Neurological Disorders and Stroke (NINDS) rt-PA Stroke Study Group. Tissue Plasminogen Activator For Acute Ischemic Stroke, New England Journal of Medicine, Dec 14, 1995, Vol 333 No. 24;1581-1587

Kay R, Wong KS, Yu YL, Chan YW, Tsoi TK, Ahuja AT, Chan FL, Fong KY, Law CB, Wong A, Woo J. Low Molecular Weight Heparin For the Treatment Of Acute Ischemic Stroke, The New England Journal of Medicine, Dec 14, 1995, Vol 333 No. 24; 1588-1593

Bukata RW. Thrombolytic Therapy for Strokes, Part I, Emergency Medical Abstracts, Nov 1996, Vol 20 No 11; 1-7

Hoffman JR. Thrombolytic Therapy for Strokes, Part II, Emergency Medical Abstracts, Dec 1996, Vol 20 No. 12; 1-7

TPA For Acute Stroke Algorithm, St. Joseph's Hospital, Huntingburg, IN, presented at Medical Staff Meeting Nov 19 1998

Caplan LR. Stroke Thrombolysis: Growing Pains, Mayo Clin Proc Nov 1997, 72:1090

Von Kummer R, et al, Acute Stroke: Usefulness of Early CT Findings Before Thrombolytic Therapy, Radiology Nov 1997, 205: 327

Tilley BC et al. Total Quality Improvement for Reduction of Delays Between Emergency Department Admission and Treatment of Acute Ischemic Stroke, Neurol Dec 1997, 54 (12):1466

Thrombolytic Precautions/TPA algorithm and protocol/National Institute of Health (NIH) "stroke scale", as printed by Memorial Hospital and Health Care Center, Jasper IN, based on outline from Indiana University Dec 1997

Bonoczk P, Gulyas B, Adam-Vizi V, Memes A, Karpati E, Kiss B, Kapas M, Szantay C, Koncz I, Zelles T, Vas A. Role of Sodium Channel Inhibition in Neuroprotection: Effect of Vinpocetine, Brain Research Bulletin, 2000,Vol 53 No. 3, 245-254

Schuchmann JA. *Stroke Rehabilitation.* Minimizing the Functional Deficits, Postgrad Med Nov1983;74(5):101-11

Rosenberg CH, Popelka GM., Post-Stroke Rehabilitation: A Review of the Guidelines for Patient Management, Geriatrics, Sept 2000 Vol 55 No. 9;75-81

Tannenbaum A, Steckly MA, Geris S. Helping Patients Resume Daily Activities After a Stroke, AJMS, January/February 2001, 36-40

Caronna J., Cerebrovascular Diseases, *Textbook of Internal Medicine,* third edition, 1997, edited by William N. Kelley, Chapter 436, 2378-2384

Dalsing MC, Lalka SG, Sawchuk AP, Mohler ER. Cerebrovascular and Upper Extremity Arterial Disease, *Textbook of Internal Medicine,* third edition, 1997, Chapter 89; 473-476

Fogleman AM, Edwards PA, Murphy FL. Pathogenesis of Atherosclerosis, *Textbook of Internal Medicine,* third edition, 1997, chapter 16, 90-94

Bennet JS. *Thrombotic Disorders, Textbook of Internal Medicine,* third edition, 1997, chapter 241; 1426-1431

Hathaway Dr. *Vascular Biology, Textbook of Internal Medicine,* third edition, 1997, chapter 14; 66-76

Jesty J, Nemerson Y. The Pathways of Blood Coagulation, *Williams Hematology,* 5th edition, 1995, Chapter 122;1227-1235

Ware AJ, Coller BS. Platelet Morphology, biochemistry, and Function, *Williams Hematology,* 5th edition, 1995, Chapter 119;1161-1191

Jaffe EA. Vascular Function in Hemostasis, *Williams Hematology,* 5th edition, 1995, Chapter 125;1263-1267

Kraft GH, Odderson IR, Halar EM. Physical Medicine and Rehabilitation, Clinics of North America, Nov 1999,10:4

Morgenstern LB. Stroke, Neurologic Clinics, May 2000 18:2

Netter FH. Volume 1, Nervous System, CIBA Collection of Medical Illustrations

Guyton AC, Hall JE. *Textbook of Medical Physiology,* tenth edition, WB Saunders 2000

Rabbi Nosson Scherman, Rabbi Meir Zlotowitz, Rabbi Sheah Brander. The Complete ArtScroll Siddur, Mesorah Publications, ltd.

Stern C, editor. Liturgy Committee of the Central Conference of American Rabbis, Gates of Repentance, The New Union Prayerbook for the Days of Awe, New York, 1978, revised 1996

Knobel PS, editor. *Gates of the Seasons,* A Guide to the Jewish Year, Central Conference of American Rabbis, New York, 1983

Stern C, editor. *On the Doorposts of Your House,* Central Conference of American Rabbis, New York, 1994

Pool DS, editor, *Book of Prayers,* 2nd edition, Union of Sephardic Congregations, 1992

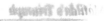

— To Order —

Matilda's Triumph
A Memoir
by Richard Moss, M.D.

If unavailable at your favorite bookstore,
LangMarc Publishing will fill
your order within 24 hours.

—Postal Orders—
LangMarc Publishing
P.O. Box 90488
Austin, Texas 78709-0488
or call 1-800-864-1648
Order from LangMarc's secured website
www.langmarc.com

Matilda's Triumph
USA: $18.95 + $3 postage
Canada: $21.95 + $5 postage

Send _____ copies $18.95   _____
   Shipping $3 + $1 additional books   _____
   TX res. 8.25%   _____
   Amount of Enclosed: _____
Send to: _____

_____

_____

Phone: _____

Check enclosed: _____
Credit Card # _____
Expiration: _____ Code: _____